A Very Decided Preference

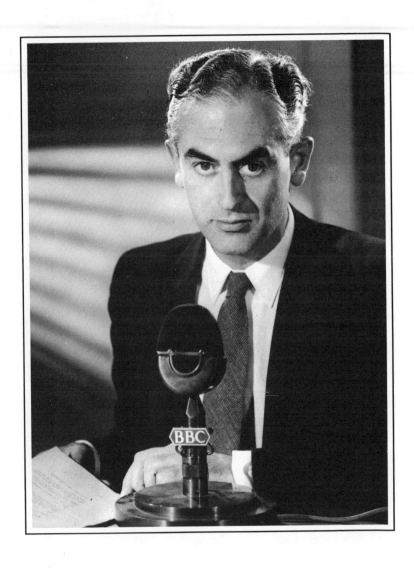

Peter Medawar

JEAN MEDAWAR

A Very Decided Preference

Life with Peter Medawar

OXFORD   LONDON   MELBOURNE

OXFORD UNIVERSITY PRESS

1990

FRONTISPIECE PHOTOGRAPH: *Peter Medawar gave six Reith Lectures on* The Future of Man *at the BBC between November 15 and December 21, 1959.*

Oxford University Press, Walton Street, Oxford OX2 6DP

Oxford New York Toronto Delhi Bombay Calcutta Madras Karachi Petaling Jaya Singapore Hong Kong Tokyo Nairobi Dar es Salaam Cape Town Melbourne Auckland

and associated companies in Berlin Ibadan.

Oxford is a trade mark of Oxford University Press.

British Library Cataloguing in Publication Data
Medawar, Jean
   A Very Decided Preference.
   1. Great Britain. Science. Medawar, P.B. (Peter Brian),
   1915–1987
   I. Title
   509.2

ISBN 0-19-217779-6

Printed in the United States of America

For our grandchildren,
born and adopted,
Benjamin, Siiri and Peter
Alexander and Theo
Flora
Anna, Toby and Daniel

For our grandchildren,
born and adopted,
Benjamin, Siiri and Peter
Alexander and Theo
Flora
Anna, Toby and Daniel

Contents

Preface

PETER MEDAWAR and I were married for fifty years. We met when we were undergraduates at Oxford. Peter was a year ahead of me, an impressive, clever, slightly farouche young man, very different in appearance from what he later became.

I realised quite soon that he was extraordinary, and exceptional. Before long others recognised this, and by the time Peter began his life's work in immunology, his quality had become apparent. He was a professor at thirty-two, a Fellow of the Royal Society at thirty-four, and a Nobel Prizewinner at forty-five.

At the height of his powers, at fifty-four, Peter Medawar suffered a terrible stroke and nearly died. Instead, he gradually recovered and lived another eighteen years, greatly handicapped but essentially unchanged in character. During these years he planned research and experiments, wrote seven more books, travelled, lectured and enjoyed life, almost in his old way. He had lost half his eyesight, the use of his left arm, and he walked with the help of a stick and a heavy splint on his left leg.

Although he suffered further major strokes in 1980 and 1985, he remained cheerful and delighted friends, colleagues, and everyone who met him with his wit and even joie de vivre. He came to be admired as much for his courage after these strokes as he had been for his intellect before them. His answer to anyone who queried his pleasure in a life with such handicaps was, ''I have a very decided preference for remaining alive.''

This book is a sketch of our life together. One of the strongest bonds between us was a belief in the hope of progress. This belief sustained Peter through the most arduous work before he was ill, and through the handicaps he suffered afterwards.

I wanted to write this story so that others could know what it was like to live with such a man. He gave joy and learning and laughter to his acquaintances, to his friends and family . . . and to me.

ACKNOWLEDGMENTS

I shall always be grateful to Edwin Barber for encouraging me to write this book, and to my friend Erika Dix for learning to use a word processor in order to produce it.

A Very Decided Preference

Flashback, Exeter Cathedral, 1969

T HE LAST NORMAL DAY Peter and I had together was Saturday, 6 September 1969. We were in the Cathedral town of Exeter in the south-west of England for the annual meeting of the British Association. The B.A., as it is called, is a serious association, founded in 1831 for the advancement of science and the edification of its lay membership. Each year a new president is elected, who presides over week-long meetings, addressed by scientists of different disciplines. The president is always a distinguished scientist and one able to round up the proceedings by delivering a sort of state-of-science speech which is widely reported. Peter was the president for 1969. He worked for months on his speech, and on eleven minor addresses he had to give during the course of the meetings. By the end of the week he had attended most of the lectures and

seminars, made speeches every evening, talked to reporters and
had been constantly surrounded by people wanting his opinion,
help or attention.

On Friday he delivered his presidential address, using Sir Francis Bacon's essay "On the Effecting of All Things Possible" as his
text. When he finished, there was silence for a few seconds, and
then a roar of applause which sounded as if it would never stop.

I wasn't surprised: I had burst into tears when he tried out the
lecture on me at home. I still think it the best and most splendid
statement on human aspirations that I have ever read or heard.
Peter wasn't dismayed by my reaction because he was himself
extremely moved by words.

After the lecture he should have been free to relax and enjoy its
success, but word came that a lecturer, due to speak on immunology to one of the special sections, had failed to turn up. Peter felt
obliged to stand in for him and he gave the lecture, extempore,
himself. I cursed the man—we could have done without that extra
strain. Later Peter wrote asking for an explanation, but none ever
came.

Saturday was mercifully a free day. Peter was longing to try
out the new car I had driven down from London and I was longing
for fresh air, so we decided to drive up onto Dartmoor and walk
there.

We stopped when we reached the foot of a big Tor, crowned
by granite rocks, and parked the car on the rough grass verge of
the road where there were only sheep to disturb it. Peter didn't
walk up—he bounded, pulling me up the hill with him. A few
minutes later he said, rather breathlessly, "You know, I really
think I could learn to like walking." This remark was music in my
ears. Hitherto, he had classified walking as boring, and made his
size his excuse. "This is what it feels like to be me," he would say,
implausibly, pressing his hands down on my shoulders. I said that
his feet were more than twice the size of mine, so . . .

We soon climbed to the top of the rocks to look down on the coloured patchwork of fields and hedges spread out below. For once, he really looked. Normally, I used to pull his arm and say, "Look, Peter, *do* look," and then he would glance at whatever it was rather than look, would smile at me and say, "Yerss—lovely," and go back to thinking. It was cool on the Tor, but we got warm running back down the hill to the car—the sheep hadn't noticed it. They were grazing the short grass on the other side of the narrow road. We explored beyond it and them and found a branch of the River Dart which had bent and scoured out a deep pool of peaty water, the colour of China tea. It was overhung with dense alder trees and a small pebbly beach ran below the bank.

I have a frequent longing to be in water—sea, river, pool or bath. We decided to bathe, there was no one around for miles; I plunged into the pool and came up gasping. I felt I was being frozen into the position of a swimming frog and I was out again in seconds. Peter thrashed around vigorously, loving it, and when he came out he said, "That was wonderful. I feel much better. We must come back tomorrow after the service and do it again." Ever since Thursday, when I had joined him at the Judges' Lodgings in Exeter, he had been tense, with an energy which needed either release or relief. After the swim he was much more relaxed; but it didn't last long. That night he slept badly, woke early on Sunday morning and was irritable. I teased him a little and reminded him that he would be off the hook as soon as he had read the lesson in the Cathedral. I made some feeble joke. He answered quite sharply, "I'm in no mood for raillery." After that I kept quiet.

He had to put on his Doctor's robes and walk in procession with the other dignitaries to the Cathedral. Someone took a rather blurred colour photo of the scene and sent it to me weeks later. As the procession filed up the nave of Exeter Cathedral, Peter saw where I was sitting and blew me an almost invisible kiss, to make up for the irritability. I guessed he must be feeling better and might enjoy reading the lesson where it would echo up into the stone fan vaulting of the Cathedral roof.

Most of the large congregation were British Association members. Traditionally, the president of the Association reads the lesson, and because Peter's speaking voice was well known and well liked this reading was much looked forward to. The Dean had proposed a passage for him to read; Peter told me that it was all about a battle, in which "the bowels of the Israelites were strewn all over the field" and, it went on—he alleged—"they gathered up of the remnants five basketsfull." He had turned down this proposed reading as having little or nothing to do with the aims and objects of the British Association. He chose instead a passage from Chapter 7 of the Wisdom of Solomon—fitting and beautiful.

At the appointed time in the service Peter rose from his seat in the Cathedral stalls, and walked to the lectern. It was the last time I saw him walk without difficulty. He began to read the lesson in a firm and well-articulated voice which carried throughout the Cathedral:

May God grant that I speak with judgement and have thoughts worthy of what I have received, for he is the guide even of wisdom and the corrector of the wise.

I began to feel easy and to enjoy his reading.

> For both we and our words are in his hand,
> as are all understanding and skill in crafts.

That fitted the modesty of good scientists.

> For it is he who gave me unerring knowledge of what exists to
> know the structure of the world and the activity of the elements.

The chemists and crystallographers might be enjoying this.

> The beginning and end and middle of times
> the alternations of the solstices and the changes of the seasons
> the cycles of the year and the constellations of the stars,

> the natures of animals and the tempers of wild beasts
> the powers of spirits and the reasonings of men
> the varieties of plants and the virtues of roots.
> I learned both what is secret and what is manifest

By now Peter began to look tired. I longed for tomorrow, and the chance to swim in the river again.

> For Wisdom, the fashioner of all things, taught me,
> for in her there is a spirit that is intelligent, holy,
> unique, manifold, subtle, mobile, clean, unpolluted,
> distinct, invulnerable, loving the good, keen, irresistible,
> beneficent, humane, steadfast, sure, free from anxiety,
> all powerful, overseeing all, and penetrating through all spirits
> that are intelligent and pure and most subtle.

He started to read more slowly. Gradually he spoke as if the words were costing him a colossal effort.

> For wisdom is more mobile than any motion;
> because of her pureness she pervades and penetrates all things . . .

Then the voice began to change and slur. Perhaps something had gone wrong with the microphone or the amplifier? It did not seem possible that anything had gone wrong with him. But it had. With horror, I guessed that he was having a stroke.

Draggingly, he finished the passage, a verger came forward and with great difficulty supported Peter as he stumbled towards his seat, gradually slumped over to the left and became unconscious. Then I *knew* that he was having a stroke. I climbed through the pews to him and helped the group of men who supported his limp body down the nave. Someone rang for an ambulance, it came, we left for the hospital and the service continued.

I had dreaded something like this for years.

It didn't seem possible to me that any machine could be always driven as Peter drove himself. He diagnosed the source of the drive as a mixture of creativity, duty, hubris and kindness—kindness because he so often obliged requests for help in writing a scientific paper or for recommendations or advice. But when I urged the need to relax, he invariably protested that, for him, a change of work was a rest. So I never saw him idle or relaxed. Now, within a few minutes, he had fallen from a pinnacle of achievements into a state very near to death.

Our life could never be the same again.

TWO

Oxford, 1935

I SAW PETER for the first time on his twentieth birthday. He was sitting on one of the hard bench seats of the zoology lecture theatre in Oxford as I came in for my first lecture. Most of his six foot four inch length was in his legs, so I didn't see how tall he was until he stood up at the end of the lecture and said to some friends sitting behind him, "Well, boys, now I'm out of my teens." He was not the kind of conventionally dressed young man I'd been used to at home in Cambridge. He wore a cheap jacket from Montagu Burton, a chain store, and a shirt of bright blue "locknit"—useful because it needed no ironing. His hair was black and curly and there was a lot of it. When he was thinking he twiddled the front part absent-mindedly, making twists which he forgot about. They made him look mildly diabolical.

During the lecture most people took copious notes. Peter scrib-

bled a word or two, crumpled up the paper and threw it away at
the end of the hour. Someone asked him why he didn't keep his
notes. "Because it's all in the textbooks," he said, and so it was. I
don't know why I still went on taking notes, but I did and so did
most of us, like sheep.

During practical work in the laboratory we dissected dogfish,
learnt to cut sections of preserved material and to identify under
the microscope various objects prepared for us on glass slides.
Often we hadn't the faintest idea what we were looking at, and the
demonstrators had to come round and explain what we were meant
to be seeing. Fortune doesn't favour only the prepared mind—the
eye also needs preparation before it can see what is there to be
seen. There was not a lot of talk in the lab, because there was
plenty to do, but we gradually got to know something about each
other, even though first-, second- and third-year students were all
mixed together. I used to hear Peter, who was in his second year,
as he towered over some student bent over his Petri dish, saying in
a mock menacing way, "Give us a fag." Some people preferred a
cigarette to the smell of formalin, dogfish or fresh rabbit insides.
Peter had a reputation for writing good and clever essays, such as
we were supposed to write for our tutors each week. I rather
wanted to borrow one of them, and mentioned this to my neighbour at the work bench. This student was a nice, orthodox young
man and he seemed to think I needed protection. He surprised me
by saying, "I suppose you've heard he's not English—he's got
Arab blood, you know," as though warning me of some danger.

When we were neither in the lecture theatre nor in the dusty
Ruskin-designed museum full of pickled or stuffed animals, or the
laboratory, we sat in the library, reading material for our essays. I
had to read a book by the philosopher J. H. Woodger and found it
very difficult. The word "heuristic" puzzled me and I couldn't find
it in the dictionary. I decided to ask Peter, who had a reputation
for knowing about philosophy. I went to where he was sitting and

asked him in a whisper to explain the meaning of the word. He did, and I thought I understood, but after a few minutes I had forgotten the meaning. I felt a fool but I thought that seeking after truth was a more important quality in a student of biology than minding about exposing ignorance, so I went back to him and confessed that I could not remember his explanation. He was very kind and this time I remembered it because he whispered that the word "heuristic" came from the Greek *Eureka* meaning "I have found it."

Later on he came to my seat in the lab and asked if I would like him to give me a few tutorials on philosophy. At this time I was more naïve than any student would now believe possible—I thought philosophy was a kind of useful, secular religion; so I accepted, and we made an appointment to meet in his lodgings at 197 Iffley Road. Peter started me with some elevated and beautiful passages from Nietzsche. I can't remember them well but they were about *die Luft der Höhe*—the air of the heights—and the heights Nietzsche was writing about were not mountainous but intellectual. Peter's choice of starting material was right, because the passage acted on me like the opening of a magic casement, through which I saw a marvellous world about which I knew nothing and he knew a great deal.

The other phrase I remember was *die Einsamkeit ist ungeheuer; das Eis ist nah*—The loneliness is awful; the ice is near. So it was lonely and cold on these intellectual heights, and I began to wonder if Peter, so different from the other young men, was lonely and cold too.

He clearly had very little money. He told me that a tramp had recently begged him for a tanner* because "I'm walking on the soles of my feet, guv'nor." Peter remembered that he had repaired the holes in his own shoes with pads of newspaper, so he gave him

---

* Slang for a coin worth sixpence (about 16 p. or 10¢).

the tanner and said, "So am I." He drank quantities of green tea, smoked odd-smelling cigarettes (his landlady thought it might be opium), and ate mainly what he could fry in a pan, over a gas ring, often cheap pats of minced meat and herbs called faggots. I had never known anyone who was not quite comfortably off and I found his scholarly pursuits and wide interests enormously attractive. Fifty-five years later—as I re-read George Eliot's *Middlemarch* to Peter—I could recognise some of those feelings in the character of Dorothea Brooke, dazzled by what she saw in the apparently intellectual Mr. Casaubon. The difference was that Peter's intellect and his character actually were as great as I guessed, only more so.

A few weeks before the final examination Peter asked, "Would you like me to get a First?" I said of course I would, and he began a very well planned scheme of revision to prepare himself for the final examination. His plan was based partly on cutting out subjects which were unlikely to be set in the final examination in June, partly by mastering subjects zoologists would have to know something about, and partly by reading up on subjects about which he already knew a great deal. He had only about seven weeks to "cram" in, but he did it, and earned a First-class honours degree.

By this time, without deep discussions, doubts or a proper proposal, he knew he wanted to spend his life with me, and I wanted to spend mine with him. I was slow to realise many things about him, and no wonder, because he was unique. He was, for instance, without any experience of what used to be called the "niceties" of life—like conventional politeness, clean clothes (his jacket was a bit smelly), and thank-you letters—and this might have put me off. I only knew that he was an uncut diamond, packed with light and fire, and I wanted to be with him permanently. I still have no idea how I recognised his quality. Later on it became obvious and everyone saw it.

I had silly ideas that we must first test whether or not I was as good as he romantically believed. To do this, I thought that something I had heard about called "inhibitions" should be removed; accordingly I proposed to drink alcohol until I could not continue with a piece of sewing I was doing and then my true nature would be revealed. Peter bought a bottle of sherry. As I was in the rather self-conscious habit of drinking milk at sherry parties (I weighed only about 8 stone* and had tuberculosis in my first year at Oxford), I had to stop sewing after my third small glass. In the middle of the fourth I felt very ill and my inhibitions were sufficiently removed to allow me to be sick into Peter's frying pan. I remember admiring his presence of mind. There would not have been time to get me to the bathroom on the lower floor. I went on feeling ill and Peter sent for a taxi to take me back to Somerville. As we climbed down the stone steps to the street, I felt I was weaving and did not want the taxi driver to think I was incapable. To show him that I was in a normal state I asked Peter, "Shall I make a remark?" As far as I can remember Peter's advice was to keep extremely quiet, but in spite of taking the advice I was again very sick when I got back to Somerville College. I don't know what all this taught Peter about me but it taught me that he could be relied on in a crisis— and his subsequent teasing convinced me that my remark would not have fooled any taxi driver for a moment.

When my father became very ill, Peter drove me home to Cambridge, in the first of his series of second-hand cars. This one had cost £5 (about $8). I didn't introduce him to my mother because I knew how unsuitable a match he would look to her, especially at that time of my father's last illness. He died in 1936, at fifty-three, worn out by repeated attacks of bronchitis. I loved him, but until he died I had not realised how much I would miss him.

It was one thing to decide to marry and quite another to achieve it. My aunt cut off the allowance she had made me, on the grounds

---

* 112 pounds.

that Peter had neither money nor "background." On learning that
Peter's father had been born in the Lebanon, my mother warned
me of the danger of having coloured babies. So did our housekeeper who, having lived in South Africa, felt she knew what she
was talking about. I protested that the Lebanese were not black,
that Peter's father had been born in Syria, and that it was in that
part of the world that Christ had been born. "That, dear," she said,
"was *very* different."

A well-known writer told a friend of my father's, when she
heard of my intended misalliance, that I would not be "received
into society." The older of my two sisters objected on the grounds
that Peter wouldn't know how to behave in a restaurant. Another
friend of my father's, a doctor who should have known better,
offered to treat a small wound on Peter's elbow in the Royal Free
Hospital. There he tested him for syphilis and even demonstrated
the sore as a chancre to medical students, though he well knew
that all the tests had been negative. This man then told me solemnly that Peter and I should not kiss. I paid no attention, collected
Peter from the hospital and drove with him back to the Pathology
Laboratory in Oxford to consult Professor Howard Florey, his
chief, who at once arranged for a bacteriological test. It showed of
course that the trouble was caused by a common infection. Peter
had caught his elbow on a dirty nail while whizzing down the
wooden tower of the helter-skelter with his young sister Pamela at
the annual St. Giles' fun fair in Oxford. Then he had gone to swim
in the public swimming baths and must have picked up bacteria
which the chlorine had been unable to subdue. With ordinary care
the wound soon healed. I found it hard to forgive my father's
friend. I had always thought the friendship was one-sided, and if
my father had been alive, I think the unethical behaviour would
have ended it.

Some time after Peter had taken his degree, his old tutor John

Young arranged an interview for him with Professor Florey (co-discoverer of penicillin and then head of the Pathology Laboratory in Oxford). Peter wanted to use tissue-culture techniques to solve a number of problems in developmental physiology—particularly one in which the growth of certain cells was inhibited by an unknown substance found in extracts of malt. This wasn't merely of academic interest; anything that promoted or checked the growth of cells might turn out to be useful in tackling the problems of cancer. Such practical possibilities always inspired him. At this stage he had a mild contempt for what he termed life-long "Studies on Variations in the Mouthparts of *Thysanoptera*," a genus of insect. Later on he vigorously defended so-called pure research, illustrating the unpredictable nature of discovery by imagining how a project designed to find a way to "make flesh transparent" would never have got off the ground—whereas X-rays were discovered by Roentgen in the course of his studies on cathode rays.

Peter called the space Professor Florey allocated to him a "handsome room, much too good for a beginner." Florey must have observed the rough diamond quality, because, as Peter later wrote, at this time, as far as research was concerned, he "had not a clue how to start." His training as a zoologist had left him totally unqualified to undertake many of the techniques he would need to use in tissue culture while searching for the unknown growth inhibitor. But he was fired by the problem, read up on the necessary techniques, and soon mastered them.

I took my degree a year after Peter and was taken on by Professor C. H. Waddington at the Strangeways Laboratory in Cambridge, in order to learn how to culture tissues. I managed to be useful and he kindly added my name to the paper he was writing. This move enabled Peter to say to Professor Florey, who asked him if he knew anyone who might be able to use tissue-culture techniques to investigate the development of lymphocytes, "Well, as a matter of fact I do." Florey asked, "Will he want a lot of money?" "No," said Peter, "as a matter of fact, I'm going to marry her."

Gradually my mother relented and let me invite Peter home; before long, and with misgivings, she generously gave me the equivalent of the allowance her elder sister had withdrawn. Peter was not capable of charming her deliberately because their interests were too far apart and nobody had taught him the sort of worldly politeness which would have reassured her, but she came to see him through my eyes. Fortunately, he developed a high temperature during his visit and had to go to bed; there he lay prone, looking and feeling rotten. This brought out my mother's kindest instincts and she stood by his bed, anxiously stroking his forehead. I could see that this was not soothing Peter, as intended, but I knew it was all for the best so I whispered, "Stick it!" and when my mother had left the room, he thought the situation so funny that he laughed himself almost better.

Peter's family made up for the disapproval I had from mine. His mother—"Mama"—never disapproved of anyone, and she welcomed me with open arms. Her sister Phyllis was much more critical, but she told Peter and he told me, that she had said to him, "Clever as you are, the cleverest thing you've done so far is to get that girl to marry you." Pamela, Peter's sister, was still at Queen Anne's School in Caversham, not far from Oxford, but in spite of the age difference we became lifelong friends. Peter's father sent me a beautiful aquamarine ring from Rio, far too grand to wear, but great to keep to look at and admire in its box.

Our two backgrounds were so different that I don't think anyone could have predicted the match. Peter was the second son of a marriage between Nicholas Medawar, a Lebanese businessman, and Edith Muriel Dowling, a very large, plain and quite wonderful English mother to whom he was as devoted as she was to him. His father ran a small business in Rio de Janeiro, called the Optica

Inglesa, and exported crystals to Zeiss in Germany. His mother decided, wisely, Peter wrote, that he, his brother Philip and sister Pamela should be educated in England rather than Brazil, so he did not have a sheltered early home life. He and Philip went to an ill-run preparatory school in Hampshire. This soon collapsed—and no wonder, for it was started by an amiably incompetent Church of England clergyman who took to the bottle, partnered by a bogus "Captain" Durgan who made off with the negotiable assets. The next step was a prep school in Broadstairs. There the headmaster was a religious maniac who got the boys to give up half their pocket money for some High Church cause; but there was also a language master called Mr. Wood who taught English and French grammar the hard way. He wouldn't have known how to conduct a conversation class, but he taught the boys grammar, how to write a précis and to read French fluently. Peter always felt grateful to him.

At the end of this period of preparation for the rigours of public school (Marlborough College), Peter had had enough outlandish experiences to hurt the most tender character. He told me once that at the Broadstairs school the headmaster had sat on his bed to confide in him that he was at risk from the attentions of the housekeeper, who, he said, was after him with a meat chopper. Peter believed that, because he had been unaffected by such events, all children were enormously adaptable and able to shrug off most peculiarities of adult behaviour. The fact was that with Philip for company, his own high spirits, vivid imagination and a headful of reading, he was better equipped than most to manage.

In Peter's early life his intellect had far more exercise than his emotions. His childhood in Rio and boyhood at school in England left no dark memories. He made fun of situations that might have hurt a different character, shouting with laughter as he told me about the rapacious housekeeper.

He read compulsively—motoring magazines, Ernest Benn's

sixpenny booklets about Stars, the Earth and Atoms, the *Strand Magazine, Tidbits and Answers,* P. G. Wodehouse, Sherlock Holmes, and Arthur Mee's *Children's Encyclopaedia.*

What he chose to read in the *Encyclopaedia* were articles that dealt with the Second Law of Thermodynamics, and Lord Kelvin's views on the probable Heat Death of the Universe. At the end of the Heat Death article, Peter noticed a faded photograph of Professor Bickerton, captioned: "Professor Bickerton, who believes that the universe is constantly renewing itself." "I bet he's right," Peter said, sanguine from an early age. What he read was processed by a superb memory, and edited with an ebullient sense of humour. At night in the school dormitory he invented stories for the other ten-year-old boys. He let them choose what sort of story it was—either an exciting drama or a comedy—and he made each instalment complete instead of part of a serial. Otherwise the boys might never have got to sleep.

Peter was a devoted son and a good and affectionate older brother to his sister Pamela and their cousin Stella. During school holidays he entertained them with stories and a hand-written newspaper called *The Pam and Stella Weekly.* In later life he was ruthless about not keeping such juvenilia. He classified them as "a farrago of clichés from low-grade detective fiction," and damned them as "completely devoid of merit." I once found him tearing up such literature and I half admired his unsentimental resolution; but I salvaged an exercise book written when he was twelve, on Astronomy, carefully composed and hand-written with a steel nib and coloured chalks—it was exemplary. He decorated the purple paper cover of the ordinary exercise book, wrote the title "Astronomy" in large letters, condensing all he had read about astronomy into chapters and sections. He threw away similar exercise books on cars and rejoiced in having made more space. I regret not having salvaged more, but Peter was very sure that "clearing out old stuff" was the right thing to do, and when he was very sure, it was difficult for me to consider that he might be wrong.

In the long holidays he went to stay with his mother and father in Rio de Janeiro. There his father started Peter's love of opera by giving him a season ticket to the opera house. The opera was well endowed and able to import superb singers from Europe. Peter used to recount their names with pleasure: Carlo Galeffi, Meta Sine-Meyer, Bidou Sayaō and Rosa Ponselle.

He learnt to play bridge with Mama and her friends, he read voraciously, played with Pamela, swam and dived through the huge rollers on Copacabana beach and gambled at the casino. Peter's father looked grave when Peter proudly showed him his wallet full of winnings, and said it would not reflect well on him as a member of the local chamber of commerce if his son were seen haunting the casino late at night. Peter pointed out that "it was one thing to have a son who lost all his money at the casino and came back for more, but quite a different thing—and not at all likely to bring discredit on him—if his son was seen to be leaving the casino with a self satisfied smile and perhaps even an air of affluence."*

The shorter holidays weren't so glamorous; a cousin called Winnie Mayger looked after Peter in Mama's rather dark basement flat in West Hampstead. It had one distinction: mixed in the gravel of the garden path were stones of rough uncut topaz, aquamarines and amethysts. Peter's father had sent home crates of these semi-precious stones. Some of the better ones were occasionally sold to Liberty's to be made into necklaces, but this trade wasn't brisk; meanwhile the weather gradually ruptured some of the crates, the stones spilled out into the garden and became a very unusual path.

Winnie was the daughter of a relation, a cousin of Mama's once removed—"not quite far enough removed," Peter used to say. Winnie's father Jack was referred to as a "ne'er-do-well," who

---

*P. B. Medawar, *Memoir of a Thinking Radish* (London: Oxford University Press, 1986), p. 100.

tried and failed at a number of ways of earning a living. When his bills mounted higher than his resources, the family did a "flit" and disappeared overnight. Consequently, Winnie's education was sporadic. She was thin, very nervous and full of fourth-hand beliefs which became family treasures. She believed that a woman's hair was her "crowning glory," but also that water rotted it, so she hardly ever dared to wash it. On kettles, her opinion was, "It doesn't do a kettle any good to go boil, boil, boil," and on fame, "It doesn't do him any good to sit back on his laurels." I never heard any family talk about Winnie that didn't close with "Poor Winnie!"—and she was poor, because she had known real poverty as well as insecurity. One day I saw her ironing, and her face looked different—she had removed her false teeth to save wearing them out. Peter told me that at the same time she would wear out her shoes, searching for food bargains in the shops of West Hampstead.

She was afraid of the dark and Peter caught this fear from her. Kind though she was, she relished frightening stories of ghosts and murders in the dark. Peter's sanguine temperament fortunately survived Winnie's care and he didn't blame her for the night terrors he had to surmount.

Holidays when Mama could return to London were different. She loved musical comedies and he was coming to love opera, so they shared a varied diet and constantly amused each other. Peter began his collection of records—most of them recordings of great singers of the past, Wilhelm Rode, Schlussnus, Rosa Ponselle, Frieda Leider, Elizabeth Rethberg and Meta Sine-Meyer among them. Years later, when he could afford to buy a complete recording of Wagner's *Ring* cycle, he told me how he had felt when he was able to buy only one record at a time. He had saved until he could afford to visit His Master's Voice shop in central London. He set out from the Greencroft Gardens flat "in a state of breathless excitement." On arrival he was allowed to choose six records to play in one of the sound-proof cubicles. He savoured every bar of the music and at last chose one to take home and play over and over on his portable wind-up gramophone. He chose well and in time this collection of his "Golden Oldies" became valuable. Years later he transferred the music onto tapes and sold the records for a price which covered the cost of a system for playing the tapes.

I was the survivor of twins and the eldest of three daughters, the family of my frail doctor father, Charles Henry Shinglewood Taylor, and my half-American mother, Katherine Lesley Paton. Her mother had died when she was four, so she was brought up by her sister Mary, twenty years older than herself. This aunt of mine, nicknamed "Tatan," was dominant and intelligent but quite ignorant of the world outside her small circle. Her parents had left her a house, and a comfortable fortune, made by her father in the cotton trade between Liverpool and Washington. At a time when she was living in a freehold house with a staff of gardener, cook, kitchen maid, bootboy, parlour maid, two house maids and a daily charlady, she once lectured me on the importance of saving money. "If I had a hundred pounds," she declared, "I would save half." She greatly influenced my mother, and I wonder whether my mother's late marriage at thirty was somehow because Tatan, who never married, did not want to lose her life's occupation.

My father hinted that she had not made it easy for him to woo and marry my mother. When he did succeed, Tatan then ran a large house in Cheshire for my Uncle Allan and he did not manage ever to marry, though I know he tried. Although Tatan tried to stop me marrying Peter, I do owe her my education at Oxford because she generously paid for it; she taught me the names of wild flowers and she also saw to it that my mother always bought shoes a little too big so that my feet were not cramped. Once I had defied her, married and had a baby, I became quite fond of her.

She should have had a university education and a job instead of having to be a mother to my mother, with no real outlets for her energy.

My mother had gone to boarding school at St. Andrew's in Scotland and there an ear infection led to an operation which left her very deaf; she learnt to lip read and she never complained about her deafness, though she once told me that she heard a pulse and singing noises in her head all the time. Her voice was pretty and hadn't the flatness of most deaf people. Her weight varied greatly from real fatness to alarming thinness and anxious overactivity. The deafness, Tatan's dominance for so many years, probable endocrine ups and downs, and a staff to manage everything left her without much interest in the world outside her home. I can remember overhearing Miss Kiddle, a governess I liked very much, say to Mrs. Pearson, who lived with us and gave us piano lessons in the not-much-used drawing room, "Now what can we think of to *interest* Mrs. Taylor?"

I'm sure she was interested in her children, but that alone doesn't attract children. She read books from the public library, which Mrs. Pearson collected for her, also *Punch* and later on a magazine—*Woman*. She knitted, but not the sort of tough bright pullovers we liked. She made and gave away so many bed jackets that we called them the "Kindly Thoughts." I think she must have been tired and bored a lot of the time, but didn't show it, except by a lack of energy or purpose. In my teens I didn't understand how she had been handicapped—I just wished she could enjoy life.

In the 1920s when I was growing up, the pressure was always to improve and to behave properly; the idea was that praise might spoil you. I thought I was thin and plain and not worth much, until a housemaid I loved told me that my Uncle Cluny had remarked to her that I had a very sweet smile. To me this was a glorious revelation. Uncle Cluny had married Edith, one of my mother's sisters, and they lived in South Africa. He did not often visit us, but I loved it when he did, because his handkerchief smelled of eau de Cologne and he joked and smiled and seemed to enjoy himself.

In 1874 my father's father, Henry Shinglewood Taylor, was a young surgeon at Guy's Hospital in London. In the diary kept at that time he noted that he had a very small supply of chloroform and that wine was the only analgesic. He was not strong, and when he left Guy's, sunshine and sea air were recommended. He took a post as ship's doctor on a boat sailing to South Africa. There he settled in the Orange Free State, practised medicine amongst Boers, Britons and Basutos, was admired and respected and became Mayor of Ficksburg. When his son—my father—was old enough, he was sent to Rugby public school in England. From there he went to Cambridge to study medicine.

Although he stroked the Cambridge boat as an undergraduate, my father once told me that he didn't reckon he was a great oarsman; but, he added, "I can hang on, though"—so grimly that I felt he knew a lot about endurance.

The journey back to Africa was long and expensive. I got some idea of how long the separation from his family had sometimes been when my Aunt Vera, his elder sister, told me that he had arrived in Ficksburg for one holiday with a doll as her present—but she had grown into her teens since he last saw her and had put her hair up.

In 1912 my father married my mother. They had only a year together before he was swept abroad by the 1914 war against Germany. After the Armistice they lived for a short time in London. About 1922 they moved to Cambridge. Until that move, when he came into my life I had no idea what he was like, where he was or what he was doing. Until April 1989 I knew nothing about where he had been in the war years—nobody talked about them.

On April 18, our friend David Pyke rang me from Oxford, where he had bought a book called *Images of Gallipoli,* saying with some excitement, "I think I've got a surprise for you."

Before he showed me the surprise he asked if my father's initials were C.H.S.T.—initials which he had seen at Downshire Hill on one of my father's watercolours. When I said they were, he opened the book; there was a photograph of my father, thin, tired and bearded, standing outside his dugout on the Gallipoli peninsula in 1915.

The book was compiled by an Australian historian of the First World War, Dr. P. A. Pedersen, from a hundred photographs taken by my father while he was serving as a surgeon in charge of the 3rd Field Ambulance station, supporting the Royal Naval Volunteer reserve expeditionary force against the Turks. The book and its chance discovery moved me enormously. From Dr. Pedersen's introduction and his captions to the photographs I learnt about the bloody and disastrous campaign—6,000 casualties for the gain of 600 yards. My father's ambulance station was only 2,000 yards behind the battle lines—the sea prevented it from being further away—and he and the expeditionary force lived for eight months in constant danger, enduring torment from heat, flies and the shortage of water.

I learnt too that he had been mentioned in dispatches for "distinguished and gallant conduct." How I wished I had known all of this before. I suppose he had kept most of the horrors from my mother, who had been very ill, and my governess and aunts probably thought I should be sheltered too. I would rather have learnt it all.

In Cambridge he began to practise medicine at 3 Trinity Street, mainly with undergraduates and particularly those who rowed or were athletes. He became interested in the physiology of athletics and in the interaction between morale and performance.

He was very popular with undergraduates, and especially with the rowing men who developed boils on their bottoms. He advised hot baths containing "flowers of sulphur." I remembered this when the sulfonamide drugs came in and hoped he had devised the treatment himself.

When he did come into my life, I was delighted with him. He seemed much more easily amused than my mother's family was. He was slightly built (I remember his weight, 10 st 10 lb (150 pounds), because it was painted on the oar hung up in his consulting room with which he stroked the Cambridge boat), and his face was brown and finely shaped. I think he wasn't afraid of spoiling me with affection, and I responded and loved him. His younger sister, Cecily, told me that he had said to her that I was "Just what the doctor ordered," and this pleased me whenever I thought of it.

I grew up in the big comfortable house in Cambridge where the money inherited from the cotton trade, plus my father's earnings from his practice (about £2,000 a year, he told me, but only when I asked), provided a governess and the same quota of staff that Tatan had.

I remember being called "delicate" all my childhood. With the idea of fattening me up for boarding school at Benenden in Kent (I then weighed 6 st 4 lb or 88 pounds), I was given lots of butter, cream and eggs, with the result that I was often sick. A low-fat diet was later prescribed and I soon longed to drink milk. Once bidden to take a mug of malted milk to my sister upstairs in bed with a cold, I drank the top off it and felt sinful but better.

At my first school in Cambridge, which was called simply "Miss Borrer's," to my surprise, I won a prize for "all round good behaviour." I think it wasn't the top prize but it was solid—a copy of Sir Walter Scott's *The Talisman*. I was about twelve and I read it with total ignorance of its background and retain no memory of its contents except that I learnt what Crusaders were.

I went on to Benenden School in the autumn of 1932 and was lucky to be in Miss Sheldon's house. The three enterprising founders of Benenden were Miss Sheldon, Miss Hindle and Miss Bird. Forty years after I left Benenden, Miss Bird invited me to stay with her after her retirement, and I asked her how the three of them, teachers at Wycombe Abbey, had had the nerve to start a new school. "We were in the stationery cupboard," Miss Bird said, "giving out stationery—and this was extremely boring. One of us said, 'Why don't we start a school of our own?' . . . and, well, we did." The three founders had a sense of humour and enjoyed themselves, doing what they had wanted to do and doing it with intelligence and enthusiasm.

What I liked most about Benenden was its position on the edge of a village—in the marvellously beautiful Kent countryside. The south coast of Kent ends in chalk cliffs, and the English Channel and the North Sea shape the eastern shoreline. The county of Kent is often called the "garden of England" because the soil is rich, and grows wonderful apples and hops for beer making. The land must once have been forested, and as the fields were carved out of the woods, small spinneys of sweet chestnut and oaks were left over to give shelter to the orchards and pastures. Every hedge was full of life—nests of dunnocks and wrens in the upper storey and voles and hedgehogs and badgers lower down. Whenever a meadow was left fallow, the wild flowers made a wild garden of delicate Queen Anne's Lace, red and white campion, burnet, poppies, scabious, clover and marguerites.

What I didn't like was the winter wind that blew across the games field, over the Weald of Kent. It shrivelled every inch of me until I got into the school lacrosse team as Cover Point; this position involved a lot of running about and jumping to catch the hard rubber ball flung toward the goal I was helping to protect, and this warmed me up a bit.

My botany mistress, Miss Wright, encouraged me to draw flowers, and I found that I could do it and get my work marked

10/10 in red ink beside the drawing; drawing for Miss Wright was always done after washing hands, sharpening pencil, and really looking at whatever part of the flower was to be drawn. It was Miss Wright who enabled me to get a scholarship to Somerville College, Oxford. At Benenden I grew stronger, made friends, and was happy at finding I was good at something.

THREE

Marriage, 1937

A S FAR AS getting married was concerned, Peter knew he could leave the tactics to me, and I enjoyed feeling that I was freeing him for more difficult things, though it would have been more fun to have had him closely involved. I remember buying the wedding ring, to save his time. I also bought a beautiful Rodier suit to get married in (reduced from £39, which was impossibly expensive for me, to £16 in the January sale at Bradley's in London); it lasted until 1949 when it was ruined in a fire in our Birmingham house.

I began looking for somewhere to live and found a flat in Banbury Road, Oxford, for £130 a year, including rates. It had four bedrooms, a sitting room, dining room, small kitchen, a bathroom and a shared garden. We got married on 27 February 1937, the day before Peter's twenty-second birthday, in the Oxford Registry Office, with both our mothers as witnesses, and then had a sherry party for friends and family in the Banbury Road flat. Bertha, my closest school friend, helped to clear up afterwards, and stayed the night. At our golden wedding party fifty years later she would have done the same again but she had to get back to Wiltshire that evening.

We started marriage as if it was a continuation of our two years friendship. When I mildly objected to excessive hours in the lab, Peter said to me, a little pompously, I thought, though I didn't have the wit or confidence to complain at the time, "You have first claim on my love, but not on my time." It would probably have been a good idea to have pointed out that love needs time-sharing, but I didn't. I knew already that his passionate questing behaviour in research needed a great deal of time and thought, and when I learnt more about his research, I came not to grudge the time, and he was grateful.

We both had romantic feelings about marriage—we were going to trust each other, have no secrets and live happily ever after. Peter's knowledge of women was based on love for his mother and sister Pamela—both of whom had a marvellous sense of humour and were easy and capable—and on books. My experience of men was mainly formed on loving and admiring my father and on romantic friendships with the selected Cambridge undergraduates who were invited home for tea on Sundays.

Peter was good at teasing me, and I wasn't used to it, but with time I got better at teasing back. One day before we were married, he asked, "Do you want to write a novel?" "Oh no." "Do you want to tell me your dreams over breakfast?" "No." "Well, then, that's all right." As we got to know one another, Peter alarmed me by telling me that he thought it was impossible for one man and one woman always to be enough for each other, and that other romantic friendships were all right, providing that the original couple truly loved each other. This belief of his was purely theoretical; he confidently expected women who attracted him to understand that his deepest emotions and most of his time were already engaged. This was not easy for them, but his women friends mostly recovered, married and became friends with both of us.

Peter was dismissive with emotional problems because he feared they might take up time he could spend better, and anyway he wasn't much interested in them. What interested Peter was *ideas*— generally illuminating ideas about the way the natural world worked, or the way human behaviour worked, but not in particular cases, about which he said he didn't know enough. So, Pavlov's work on the conditional reflex was fascinating, but why a fellow student stole Peter's books wasn't. He did want his books back, though, so he marked one he was fairly sure would be stolen, and caught the thief—till then a friend. All the ex-friend said was, "I suppose I was a fool to try it on with you." He did not seem either sorry or ashamed and went on to have a respectable career.

I always wanted to unravel and understand any differences that upset us, though there weren't many, and often badgered Peter to pay attention, usually without success, until I got really upset. Then he would be very contrite and concerned and we would be what he called "greatest friends" again. Our strongest bond was a hopeful attitude to life, faith in what science might achieve, and a deep commitment to each other. The French poet and airman St. Exupéry wrote, "Love is not gazing forever into each other's eyes, but looking in the same direction." We were polarised to look in the same direction, and we saw both the same and different views. Peter once told me that he felt he would have had a nervous breakdown if his energies had not been channeled into science and if he had not found a lifelong companion who understood and loved him.

The day after we married, we went together to the Sir William Dunn School of Pathology for the first time. As we walked up the rather grand steps, one flight on each side of the double doors, we met Miss Campbell-Renton, one of the staff who knew Peter. "Hello," she said, "won't you introduce me?" I expected Peter to say, "May I introduce my wife, Jean"—it was his first chance; but instead he absent-mindedly introduced me as Miss Taylor.

In the spring of 1937 we were invited to Potsdam for a short holiday by the German Jewish parents of a young man whom we had met the year before. Louis Hagen, nicknamed Büdi, was the second son of the head of one of the last private banks in Germany. Büdi was high-spirited and careless. One day, away from home in Potsdam, aged about seventeen, he wrote a postcard to his sister and rashly allowed himself to add a rude remark about Hitler. A housemaid, under notice for stealing his mother's jewellery, found and read it. If she was dismissed, she told Frau Hagen, she would report Büdi to the police. Büdi's parents bravely told her to leave, she informed, and Büdi was arrested.

The prison he was taken to had been adapted from an old fortified castle. The prisoners were made to run round the court-yard until the older ones fell down, exhausted. The guards amused themselves by kicking those they particularly disliked into a shallow muddy pond within the castle walls; as each tried to crawl out, they were kicked back, until they died in the mud. All this Büdi saw, out of his barred window overlooking the courtyard. He was often singled out in the middle of the night for the brutal amusement of young guards, delighted to have an opportunity of beating up a contemporary whose life had been more privileged than theirs, and who was a Jew, one of those whom they had been taught to hate. The prisoners had to clean the latrines with their bare hands. The metal handles of the full buckets they then had to carry away took the skin off their hands and the palms became infected.

One day a big Mercedes drove through the gate of the castle. Inside was a well-known judge, the father of one of Büdi's school friends. He demanded to see Louis Hagen—he had a permit to release him. The Commandant marched Büdi to the guard house.

If he told anyone how the prisoners were treated, he said, "We will get you, wherever you are, and bring you back, and you will never get out again." Finally Büdi was driven away in the car with the judge. The two SS men sitting in front with the driver were separated from them by a glass panel. In spite of fear of being overheard or observed, Büdi showed his hands and described what went on in the castle. The judge, then a member of the Nazi Party, was appalled. He subsequently resigned his position and was banished to a small town in East Prussia. Büdi's family had influence enough to get him out and over to England, where he was found a lowly job in the Pressed Steel works in Oxford. After we got to know him, we made him an honorary member of our family and the godfather of our first child, Caroline, born in July 1938. He is now a grandfather, but is still ebullient, resourceful and kind.

The Hagens' house on the edge of a lake near Potsdam had been built for the family of five children and retainers, and had plenty of room for parties and guests. Büdi's parents were very kind to us. Büdi had warned us not to expect satisfying meals, and it was as well he did. The Hagens believed in a diet of vegetables, fruits, nuts and raisins, and this was the menu of our first meal with them. When Büdi was growing up, he and his two brothers and two sisters were each allowed only one egg a week, on the grounds that more might exacerbate their sexual appetites. The regime didn't work successfully for any of them.

Peter booked tickets for a performance of Wagner's *The Valkyrie* at the Berlin opera house. This was my first opera and a great occasion, so we dressed in our best. Both Peter and the programme described for me how the beautiful Sieglinde, married by force to the unpleasant Hunding, fell in love with Sigmund before she realised that he was her twin brother.

The music was moving—like nothing I'd ever heard. A stout lady in a sort of nightgown trotted on the stage, which depicted Hunding's hut in a primaeval forest. "Is she the Putzfrau [cleaning lady]?" I whispered to Peter. He stifled a cross between a laugh and a groan. She was Sieglinde.

Although Peter's emotions were deeply stirred by words, they were stirred even more deeply by Wagner's music. He often said that the stories in the *Ring* cycle were "all rot" but the combination of music and words in these operas affected him profoundly. Many years later he wrote that he was "spellbound by the later operas of Wagner whose gifts included the power to transport me out of the real world into one of extravagant make-believe."* As Bryan Magee wrote in *Aspects of Wagner,* "It is in the orchestra . . . that the innermost aspects of the drama are being realised. The most important things in life, namely its psycho-emotional fundamentals, as inwardly experienced, are articulated here, as they never can be in words, or on the stage, in any other outward terms. . . . Wagner's music expresses, as does no other art, repressed and highly charged contents of the psyche, and that is the reason for its uniquely disturbing effect . . . it makes possible a passionate warmth and fulness of emotion without personal relationships."†

I don't think that the highly charged contents of Peter's psyche—and it certainly was highly charged—were really stirred until he was enthralled by music, especially the music of the *Ring,* and by falling deeply in love. He used to hold my hand throughout the whole cycle, sometimes so hard that my wedding ring hurt my fingers. One of the most gripping moments in the cycle comes when Wotan bids farewell to his disobedient daughter Brunnhilde, before encircling her with a ring of protective flames. This arrangement is to ensure that the hero who will ultimately claim her should be one, as Wotan sings, "worthier than I." Years later I complained that this archetypal scene seemed to move Peter more than having to say goodbye to his own daughter when she was leaving home for months; at the time he seemed hardly to notice

---

Memoir of a Thinking Radish, p. 100.
† Bryan Magee, *Aspects of Wagner* (New York: Stein & Day, 1969), p. 66.

she had gone. "My emotions are heightened by art," he explained, but I did not find the explanation *quite* enough.

Love frustrated by misunderstanding, as in Violetta's passionate sacrificial farewell to Alfredo in Verdi's *La Traviata,* or by separation, always brought on choking emotion. When Brunnhilde announces to Siegfried that she is shortly going to gather him up to Valhalla, and without his sweetheart sister, Peter almost wanted the music to stop, he was so painfully stirred.

All I remember about Berlin was Büdi's brother Peter taking us to a nightclub; and all I remember about that was a conversation with a pleasant man, most easy to talk to. Later, Peter told me that he was a homosexual. That was interesting: until then I had imagined all homosexuals were affected, posing men who didn't like women.

When we returned to Oxford, I worked in my room next to Peter's in the Pathology Lab on the problem Professor Florey wanted tackled. The aim was to discover the function of lymphocytes. These white blood cells are manufactured in the lymph glands and are poured into the blood every day, but their numbers in the circulation do not increase. Were they, as earlier researchers Maximov and Bloom had declared, the primitive white cell from which all others developed, or had they a special function of their own? The simple work I did provided material for a thesis which I offered for a B.Sc. degree. Peter taught me about how to write a thesis and he typed it for me at tremendous speed, with two fingers. I'm not sure I would have been awarded it if he had not helped so much.

We lived simply; supper out at the City restaurant was a treat and cost only 2s.6d. each. We didn't dream of helping the three simple courses down with wine, still less of keeping a bottle in the house—until Peter's mother came to stay, six o'clock came round, and there was nothing to drink. After that we kept a bottle of something for emergencies.

When Peter was elected to a Junior Fellowship at Magdalen, he endured the ritual of being asked "to take wine" with each of the other Fellows. He came home with his eyes slewing and a bad headache. I did what I had seen done in similar circumstances in American films. I helped him to lie down on the sofa and put a towel full of ice on his forehead. It wasn't very successful because the ice soon melted, but anyway he slept—until there was a ring at the door of the flat. Two ladies I had never met appeared. "We are old friends of your mother-in-law, my dear; we were passing and just thought we'd see how you are getting on." My heart dropped, but Peter behaved beautifully, even with so little warning, and they had no cause to report back to Mama that her son had taken to the bottle and was sleeping it off.

Nearly every evening after supper Peter played his records and made adjustments to the "sound box" which he had made for his gramophone. This was the "head" that held the needle, either steel like a sewing needle or a sharp piece of bamboo which constantly had to be recut with a clipper. The gramophone had to be wound up by hand for each record and the music, mostly Wagner and Verdi, conducted by Peter, came out of an enormous trumpet; it probably resounded in the flats above and below too, but nobody complained.

I knew little or nothing about politics, but I didn't like the Conservatives' foreign policy, so I joined the North Ward of the Oxford Labour Party as its secretary, and tried unsuccessfully to get Frank Pakenham (now Lord Longford) into Parliament instead of Quintin Hogg (now Lord Hailsham). I thought that the Prime Minister, Mr. Chamberlain, understood very little if he believed that Hitler had "no further claims in Europe," as he had declared. A march was arranged in Oxford, and placards saying "Chamberlain must go" were provided. For once, I got Peter out of the lab and he marched beside me, grumbling mock seriously, "It's all very well for you down there, everybody can see me up here."

"All the better," I told him. Our marching against Chamberlain of course had no effect; Hitler invaded Czechoslovakia, and the nightmare prospect of war came closer. At one point Peter put his arms round me and said very seriously, "If I'm called up, you won't make a fuss, will you?" He always planned ahead and of course I could only answer, "No, I won't."

When war was declared in 1939, Peter was not called up. The Recruiting Board told him it was his duty to continue to teach medical students and where possible undertake research that might be "of service to the medical establishment." A contributing factor against calling him up was, he alleged, the size and flatness of his feet and his height. Size 13 boots might have been difficult to find. So he was left safely in Oxford to teach medical students, and his energy for research was further fuelled by a feeling of guilt that he was not at risk, as his contemporaries were.

In the early days of the war he sometimes played bridge in Magdalen College with the philosophy don Harry Weldon and his friends. Harry Weldon was a great figure in pre-war Oxford. Peter wrote that Harry was "a man whose speech, manners and address to life profoundly influenced all the young men who came in contact with him." Of course I never came into contact with him—there was no overlap in our lives and could have been little or no conversation. Dons in Oxford colleges then were all male and mostly unmarried, and were mildly jealous if one of their company preferred to eat with his wife at home instead of with them in college. I never met Harry Weldon, but if I had I would have recognised him from Peter's description: "He had a distinctive and distantly audible tittering laugh which he exercised continually to give an edge to or to invite concurrence with opinions which were usually comprehensively and unsparingly cynical."*

Peter had got to know him through his tutor John Young, who

*Memoir of a Thinking Radish.

had recognised and approved Peter's taste for philosophy. John arranged for Peter to take tutorials in Kantian philosophy from Harry Weldon; soon he became one of the audience when Harry felt like giving a dazzling display of epigrams and aphorisms to the young students who sat at his feet. Peter asked himself years later what was in it for the dazzler. He guessed it was "an exhilarating ego trip and the sort of exultant feeling an athlete must have after turning in a superlative performance." I know what Peter meant, but I think comparison with an actor would have fitted better; an athlete's superlative performances usually end in gasping, utter exhaustion.

Peter often wanted to go on playing bridge when the others were ready to stop. Once, late at night, he excused this urge by explaining to the other three, "My mind, you know, it never lets me rest." Harry Weldon replied coldly, "Or anyone else's."

In the summer of 1937, eight of us who had been students together decided to visit the great exhibition in Paris. We went by boat and paid a return fare of £5. We stayed in a small hotel on the Left Bank and I enjoyed everything until I ate a piece of quiche from an open air stall and thereafter spent more time looking for *cabinets de toilettes* in the imposing palaces of each nation than looking at their contents. Before we left we were drawn into a booth selling Oriental rugs. The salesman recognised the Arabic origin of Peter's name and made much of us with sweet tea and soft rugs to sit on. One orange, cream and black rug was a reasonable price and I wanted to buy it. Peter was sure we would have to pay customs duty. Our hosts promised, vehemently, that no customs officer would charge for such a small domestic rug—not for such beautiful people, and so on. I believed them, but the others didn't and teased me. I bought the rug and when we landed the English customs officer charged duty, as he was supposed to do. I was upset, not for being wrong but because I had trusted the Arabs. I wrote to their address in Morocco. I can't remember what I wrote but it must have touched them because they sent back the duty money with a charming letter in French. Peter was amused, delighted—and amazed.

Many of our friends thought the world was in far too awful a state to bring a baby into, but we preferred a more hopeful attitude to the future. In April 1938, Professor Florey noticed the strain on the buttons of my white lab coat and said dryly, "I think it's time you stayed at home, Geheimrat." He called everyone who worked with him by this honorific title, and I expect it saved him remembering our names, though he didn't forget what work we were doing. So I stayed at home and actually began knitting the small white woolly garments which were the predecessors of the easy-care stretch clothes babies now wear.

Peter loved the idea of having a family; he described it once in the biblical phrase of having "olives round my table." When a baby was born, without fault, he marvelled at the perfection of skin, tiny nails and toes; but he seemed not to feel a need to be deeply involved, for his own delight or relaxation. He *could* have learnt to put on a nappy—and in 1939 there was still some skill to it—but I don't ever remember him doing it, though if I had asked, he would have tried. He was very large and a baby is very small, and he was never sure how to hold one to make it comfortable. But in his and my father's time, fathers were not expected to know how to look after babies and young children—that was women's work—and besides the current social mores, Peter was intensely preoccupied.

Caroline was born in July 1938 at a time when Peter was finishing a series of complicated experiments, quite as time-consuming as a nursery full of children. After I came home from hospital I suggested that we both needed a holiday and he arranged to spare two weeks in August. The Spanish War was raging and we heard that children were starving in Madrid. I collected enough money, £10, to buy dried milk in France, and we were given the name of a Quaker in Perpignan who could arrange to transport it over the border.

We took Caroline and a nurse to my mother's house in Cambridge. There she was much loved and well looked after by a nurse, grandmother and staff, so I felt no anxiety for her, only relief that Peter would take a holiday and that we could do something to help the Spanish children. We packed into a baby Austin car and set off through France to find the owner of a garage in Perpignan on the French-Spanish border who was supposed to know how to arrange for the milk to get into besieged Madrid.

We took three days driving south through France and the last two were extremely hot—the Austin 7 had neither a sun-roof nor air conditioning. Sometimes we ate bread and cheese under a tree at midday and sometimes Peter unwisely drank some wine. After that, he kept on asking me to pinch him or sing to him to keep him awake. His repertoire of songs was much better than mine and for the first time I heard his schoolboy rendering of the Nile Scene in Verdi's opera *Aïda,* in which he sang the parts of both the father Amonasro and his daughter, as he had done at Marlborough with his musical friend Vincent Godefroy. We neither of us had good singing voices, but the noise kept him awake and by the end of the journey I knew Aïda's words, though I couldn't reach the high notes of her arias.

We had been assured that the garage man in Perpignan knew what he was about and would see the milk over the border and on its way to the children. When we found the man, Peter was cynically doubtful if he was reliable. I hope the milk got to the babies.

Very soon England would also be at war with Germany—a conflict for which the Spanish War had been the dress rehearsal.

FOUR

War Years in Oxford,
1939‒1945

I N SEPTEMBER 1939 a broadcast by the Prime Minister, Mr. Chamberlain, announced that we were at war with Germany. "I am speaking to you from No. 10 Downing Street," he said solemnly. "This morning the British Ambassador in Berlin handed the German Government a final note, stating that unless the British Government heard from them by 11 o'clock that they were prepared at once to withdraw their troops from Poland, a state of war would exist between us. I have to tell you now that no such undertaking has been received, and that consequently this country is at war with Germany. . . ." The hair-raising wail of a siren followed the broadcast. My heart still sinks whenever I hear that sound again. It heralded the start of an entirely new way of life.

The war came to Oxford only in the form of evacuees, food

rationing, black-out curtains and dread of what might happen if we lost. Goebbels's views on racial purity were well known through his broadcasts; Goering was liable to draw his gun, so he said, at the mention of culture—so our family, like so many others, would qualify for the Nazi firing squad. Sir Edward Grey's words in 1914—"The lamps are going out all over Europe"—described the atmosphere of the start of the Second World War just as well as the First.

In the Pathology Lab Peter had been following research ideas that might be, as the Recruiting Board had put it, "of service to the medical establishment." When he recalled this time in his memoirs some forty years later, he wrote that he thought he hadn't really "got anywhere or done anything to speak of," but he had not lost confidence in his ability to tackle scientific problems. He solved several small ones and completed a series of experiments on the effect of wounds and deep burns on skin.

At this point in the war, Professor Howard Florey and his team were urgently searching for substances which would kill bacteria without harming the body they were infecting. They decided to follow up an observation made by Professor Alexander Fleming in St. Mary's Hospital Laboratories in London. Fleming had noticed that some spores of the blue mould which grows on damp bread had infected one of his bacterial cultures growing in a dish of nutrient jelly. Where the spores had developed there was a clear area. This at last made sense of the seventeenth-century treatment which used blue mould and cobwebs as a healing poultice for wounds. This particular mould had killed off the bacteria. Fleming had also been looking for a substance which killed bacteria better than the disinfectants which had been in use since Lister's discovery that solutions of carbolic had a sterilising effect.

In 1940, anything which could be used in the treatment of war wounds was urgently needed. Accordingly Professor Florey, Dr. Ernst Chain and Dr. Norman Heatley began working to isolate pure penicillin from the blue mould. The apparatus they first designed for its extraction—stills, retorts, tubes, clamps, bungs and bottles—almost filled the central stairwell of the Sir William Dunn School of Pathology, but it worked, and they produced enough of the pure stuff to start testing its safety and efficacy.

Florey then asked Peter to find out if the extract they called penicillin was toxic to tissues. Peter cultured various tissues with different strengths of penicillin in solution and the results showed that it was not—it could be safely used on human tissues. He was proud that his name appeared in what he called the "credit titles" of the paper "Further Observations on Penicillin" published in Vol. 2 of *The Lancet* in 1941, by H. W. Florey and six colleagues.

During the first summer of the war a warning was broadcast by the Air Ministry that Oxford might be attacked in daylight by low-flying enemy bombers. The weather was wonderful that summer, and one weekend afternoon Peter, young Caroline and I were in the garden of 110 Banbury Road—Peter reading and I either minding Caroline or tending to the rows of vegetables. Suddenly we heard the approaching roar of a bomber, then saw it flying, very low, towards us through the birch trees at the end of the small garden. I picked Caroline up without thinking, and as I scrambled into our homemade air-raid shelter with her under my arm, I heard an enormous dull thump as the plane landed in Professor J. S. Haldane's garden in Cherwell Road, not far from us. The plane was English, not German, and one of the men on board was very badly burned—two thirds of his body suffered burns that had damaged the whole thickness of his skin.

Peter was asked to try to help. He visited the man in hospital and was shaken by what he saw. From then on there were no more of what he called "messing about" experiments. The greater part of his time, energy and thought immediately became devoted to finding an answer to the crucial question: how does the body discriminate between its own and other living cells, between what

Sir Macfarlane Burnet called Self and Non Self?

He worked like a demon. This was not an academic problem—lives now depended on it. Skin from one person grafted onto another was known not to survive, so Peter began to devise a means of eking out what might be spared of the patient's own skin to cover the burnt area. He tried growing small pieces of skin, left over from plastic repair operations, in tissue culture, to increase their size; he tried harvesting epidermal cells, from outer layers of skin, making them into a kind of soup and spreading them over the raw area of the patient's burn; and he tried applying extremely thin slices of skin on the wound. He found that only full-thickness skin would help, because without the dermis, or outermost layer, the wound contracted to form terrible and sometimes handicapping scars. In the end the patient was successfully treated by a Spanish surgeon, Dr. P. Gabarro, who used "postage stamp" grafts. These small pieces of skin were a compromise between the epithelial soup and the seldom available whole skin graft large enough to cover the burnt area. In this technique, cells gradually spread out between the postage stamps to form a covering of makeshift skin. Years later, in 1988, I learnt from the BBC that during research on a programme they were making about Peter they had traced the burnt airman to Canada, where he was successfully rearing Alsatian dogs.

Peter moved on to tackle the crucial problem of why skin could not be accepted by one individual from another. However carefully applied, grafts from one person to another did not take. Blood can be transfused, so why should not skin be exchanged? He asked the War Wounds Committee for support and they gave him a grant to work in the Burns Unit of the Glasgow Royal Infirmary, where both patients and facilities for research were available. He left home for two months, staying in a hotel which would now be given a pretty low star rating. At the suggestion of the bacteriologist Dr. Leonard Colebrook, he began to work with Tom Gibson, a very intelligent surgeon working in Mr. Clarke's Surgical Unit at the Infirmary. Together they decided that the first task was to find out exactly what went on inside grafts of donated skin (homografts) which made them behave differently from those taken from the patient (autografts).

Their first patient was a Mrs. McK, an epileptic whose back was badly burnt when she fell onto her gas fire. Mrs. McK was not expected to survive, but she did. She had a brother, a policeman, who volunteered to supply enough skin to provide a series of small "pinch grafts" for grafting onto the raw area of his sister's back. Alongside these grafts Tom Gibson and Peter set a parallel row of tiny (4–6 mm autografts) from Mrs. McK herself. They monitored both sets, by eye and microscopically—and here the histology classes of the zoology course came into their own. Peter prepared the samples, impregnated them with wax, sliced them into sections, stained them and studied them under the microscope. At first there was not much difference between the homografts and the autografts, but after a few days the homografts were invaded by lymphocytes—the white blood cells that spy out foreign intruders—and in about ten days they were rejected and fell off. Tom Gibson had noticed from his clinical observations that if a second set of homografts was applied at this point, they did not last long. Peter's hypothesis was that homografts were rejected in the same way as invading bacteria or foreign cells are rejected. The body couldn't be expected to "know" that the grafts of foreign, non-self skin were meant to help, and it would therefore mount the usual rejection reaction.

So, to test his guess, when the first set of grafts fell off, a second set of skin grafts from Mrs. McK's brother was applied, and then as Tom Gibson and Peter expected, they saw with excitement that this set had been at once invaded by lymphocytes and cast off much more rapidly. By now the body had been made ready to attack the foreign "antigens" brought in on the homografts, with the "antibodies" which developed on its lymphocytes in response to the first set.

In the paper they subsequently wrote, entitled "The Fate of Skin Homografts in Man" (*Journal of Anatomy,* 1943), they proposed the idea that homografts were rejected through an immunological response. This was a crucial theory, made possible by imagination, hard work and a fruitful partnership. Through it, they moved the problem into a recognised field, the field of immunology; but the hypothesis rested on only one case. So when he got back to Oxford, Peter set about substantiating it with detailed study of the phenomenon of skin homograft rejection in rabbits.

A paper, published two years later, described how he had taken six hundred grafts from twenty-five rabbits and had transplanted a graft from each onto each of the other rabbits.* He looked after the rabbits, their cages and food himself because he didn't think that the Italian prisoners-of-war detailed for the work would be careful or solicitous enough; he also cut, stained and photographed the sections of each graft himself, because there were no technicians to help, and he did this while giving tutorials that sometimes kept him from home until eleven-thirty at night. It was worth the effort: he and Tom were right. The homografts were being rejected because the body had mounted an immunological attack on them.

It was basically this discovery and all the work that flowed from it which led to the Nobel Prize over fifteen years later. Immunology—the study of the intricate means whereby the body defends itself against bacterial or other invaders—was given a great boost, and the brightest surgeons became urgently interested in the new prospects. This led to an increase in experiments to discover the mechanisms of graft rejection and ways of suppressing the im-

---

* 600 rather than 625 because a few experiments fell by the wayside.

mune response which could have clinical application. Might the
reaction be suppressed while the skin or organ grafts were supposed to be settling down in their new home?

Many years before this discovery of the nature of the host's
reaction to the donor graft was published, some surgeons had
guessed that its failure to "take" might be caused by genetic differences between donor and host, and others had even suggested that
the rejection mechanism might have an immunological basis. What
the Glasgow study on Mrs. McK did was to crystallise these ideas
and show beyond doubt that they were correct. All over the world
research developed on different aspects of the body's immune
system. Later on, in 1962, when the International Transplantation
Society was established at a congress in Paris, Peter was elected
its first president.

While Peter was working ferociously on urgent problems, my
job, like thousands of other wives' jobs, was to be a sort of life
support system. Everything possible had to be saved and nothing
wasted; this sort of frugality takes time and energy. The flat had
no central heating and nothing except a clothes line for drying
clothes and a bath tub to wash them in.

A second baby was born in 1942—called Charles after my
father and Peter after his father.

Our only form of heat was an open fire or an expensive electric
fire. At last we managed to buy a stove for the sitting room. It was
called an Otter and it burnt coal which Peter carried in bags up the
stairs. With careful raking and stoking, the Otter's fire could be
made to last all night and by morning a pile of clothes left on top
would be warm and dry, with a pleasant smell—unless the wind
changed and the draft became too much, when the smell changed
to one I dreaded, scorched cotton and the ruin of nappies.

We once ran out of coal. Word went round that a small supply
could be picked up from the goods yard of the station. As I lugged
my bag out of the yard, I saw another pile of coal from which I

could easily have added to my ration. I realised then how relative much morality is. If the children had been cold, I would have stolen, as skilfully as possible.

I worked out that, in all, I washed about five miles of nappies by hand for Caroline and then another five miles for Charles; there were then no tinned baby foods, so I puréed fresh vegetables and cooked the rations for ourselves and two girl students evacuated from the Slade School of Art in London. The Ministry of Food published good recipes to help with rations—four ounces of meat per person each week, one ounce of butter, one ounce of lard, one ounce of sugar. Dried peas, beans and lentils were available, and with potatoes, green and root vegetables, tinned or frozen fish, and a little cheese we had a healthy though boring diet. Once, whale meat appeared in the fish shops. It was red but tasted fishy and we dutifully tried it. I couldn't eat it now, knowing more about whales than I did then, unless I was starving. I don't remember feeling hungry, but when Caroline was about three she must have felt a need for fat. Once I found her sucking a cube of lard, still in its piece of grease-proof paper. She climbed from a chair, up onto a draining board beside the sink to reach the lard ration in the larder—the perforated zinc box which projected from the kitchen window and was what we had to keep perishable food in until we had a refrigerator. I sympathised with her.

Some newspapers went too far in devising economical recipes. I remember the worst was called Savoury Babas. You were advised to soak stale buns in a mixture of powdered milk and powdered eggs, to add seasonings and spicy bottled Worcester Sauce, and then bake. What really irritated me about this recipe was that on serving you were told to watch for the "expressions of delight on Daddy's face" as he tasted the buns.

As well as teaching, lecturing, research work and writing scientific papers, Peter enrolled as a fire watcher, and was briefed what to do if an incendiary bomb fell on the roof of one of the laboratories. The fire watchers had only a stirrup pump and a few buckets of sand to put out fires, which would have been hopelessly inadequate; luckily their efficacy wasn't tested. The nearest Oxford got to the experience of being bombed was the pulsating drone of the Luftwaffe's engines overhead on nights when the moon was full, on their way to bomb Coventry or Birmingham.

As part of the war effort a group of us made baby's clothes for refugees from Europe, and we mended anything mendable. We cut and sewed once a week in the house of Professor le Gros Clark in Bellbroughton Road. I made three little vests out of a pair of underpants donated by the Master of Balliol, Dr. A. D. Lindsay— a large man. Saving electricity was supposed to free more for the factories making armaments. I read the electric meter and made a graph of units used each day. A German refugee lady called Mrs. Landesberger came three times a week to help with the chores and I could always tell on which days she came because the graph soared up. In Germany she had been used to washing up under the running hot tap, and found it hard to see that giving up the practice could in any way help the country's war effort. The Nazis had wrenched rings from her hand as she left the country, so I had hoped she would save electrical units more enthusiastically than I did, but her mind did not work that way.

No. 110 Banbury Road was divided into three flats; the top flat above us was soon occupied by the Kosterlitz family, also forced to flee from Germany because they were Jews. Dr. Kosterlitz was a psychoanalyst and until he was rounded up as an enemy alien, Peter sometimes played chess with him. This entertainment was mixed with frustration by Dr. Kosterlitz's habit of asking if he could take a move back "because I have made a mistake." A fairly steady stream of patients made their way up the stairs to the top floor for treatment. Peter was already sceptical about the therapeutic value of psychoanalysis and saw and heard nothing from the top flat to change his views.

The business of raising small children and keeping a flat and garden going on rations seems tough in retrospect, but at the time it didn't, because compared with what was happening in the war zones and especially in besieged Leningrad, we were lucky. Without television, we were spared the ghastly spectacles of what war does to people. We did what we could to help the war effort and for the rest got on with what passed for ordinary life.

Peter was now twenty-nine and a university Lecturer. On 20 November 1944, an American biology graduate, Gordin Kaplan, then serving in the U.S. Army and stationed near Oxford, came to a lecture of Peter's. Afterwards he introduced himself. Peter took him on a tour of the dusty specimens in the Ruskin Museum and they began to talk. Both had tremendous ebullience, wit and irreverence, and they amused each other at once. At about six o'clock Peter came to a halt and said to Gordin, "Do excuse me, old chap, my wife is having our third child in the Radcliffe Infirmary. I must just pop over and see whether it's a boy or a girl." Gordin was already an Anglophile and understood the Oxford fashion for flippancy and understatement, and especially for treating serious subjects with apparent levity. I heard this story from him forty-four years after he heard it from Peter. What it turned out to be was a fine girl, weighing seven and three-quarter pounds, and we called her Mary Louise. Her sister Caroline and her brother Charles called her Loulie, and this pet name stuck.

I came home after the regulation two weeks in hospital (which at least gave mothers the only rest they were likely to get) and found the children coughing. The endless dry hacking turned out to be whooping cough and there were fears that the baby might catch it. So I tried not to carry whooping cough from Caroline and Charles, in bed at one end of the L-shaped flat, to the baby in a small room at the other end. This involved changing into a white coat and washing my hands each time I went from one to the other—precautions that were probably only ritually effective. The coughing lasted all winter; by the spring we decided to try the traditional cure of country air and farm food.

I found a farm called Puddle End at Northleigh, a village a few miles outside Oxford, on the edge of the Cotswolds. The lane leading to the farm was full of cow-trodden puddles and Peter looked gloomy when he saw how primitive the farmhouse was: the only heat came from a small coal fire in the sitting room; there I would have to sterilise Loulie's bottles, and the only source of hot water was a sooty kettle balanced on the same open fire. For Peter, the bottom line on the amenity scale was an outside privy, but that we were spared. On the plus side, Caroline and Charles could run out of the front door to play in the fields, pick daisies and watch, astonished, how the cows grazed and munched all day long. The hawthorn hedges were sprouting shining green leaves, the meadow grass was growing fast and white violets were starting to flower in the hedgerows.

We invited godparents and friends for Loulie's christening in the parish church. I made a wreath of moss and white violets for the font and we had a primitive party afterwards—cake made with real eggs, pots of tea and buns.

Every weekend Peter left his work in the laboratory and drove the ten miles out to see us. The children thrived on the farm food. By the end of April they had stopped coughing and we drove home, slowly, at about 28 miles an hour, to save on the petrol ration.

FIVE

The "Boy Professor," 1947–1952

WHEN PETER WAS THIRTY-TWO, he was invited to become Professor of Zoology at Birmingham University. He was pleased and a little surprised to be asked—he was not a conventional zoologist with a detailed knowledge of the animal kingdom. In fact it was well known to his students that he was unwilling to identify anything, usually because he couldn't—but if the specimen was captured in a matchbox he wouldn't, in case it was a tarantula that might have entered the country in a bunch of bananas. He was genuinely put out by spiders; if one got into the house from the garden and sat looking down at us from the ceiling, it was I who had to catch it and return it to the garden.

Peter attributed the Birmingham invitation to the machinations of Dr. Solly (now Lord) Zuckerman. He wrote: "One of his [Solly's] first thoughts on accepting the Chair of Anatomy was to contrive such other appointments as would make the University a more congenial environment for himself, and to my great satisfaction his first thought on this last score was to import me and my wife."* Solly had recognised Peter's quality from his days at Oxford, and he knew me because he was tutor for my special subject, "the social behaviour of mammals and birds with special reference to flocking." What an impossible subject for a young and uncritical girl. Peter was interviewed by Sir Norman Haworth, the Nobel Prize-winning chemist and autarch of the Birmingham University campus. If Sir Norman decided that Peter was the young man that the Department of Zoology and the University wanted as professor, his opinion was not likely to be questioned.

To start the conversation, Sir Norman handed Peter a test tube containing a few millimetres' depth of a white crystalline powder which he identified as a type II pneumococcal polysaccharide and said, "Discuss!" The crystals were part of the killing form of the bacteria which caused pneumonia. Nothing in the zoology course had prepared Peter for this, but for his own interest he had read Landsteiner's famous book on serological reactions and the dramatic story of how the mild form of the bacteria transformed into one that almost invariably killed the patient, so he was delighted to discuss the subject. After this successful interview, with the least possible delay, he was appointed to the Chair of Zoology in the autumn of 1947.

Peter's youth (Solly called him the "Boy Professor") might have been a disadvantage, but his great height and bearing compensated. By now his student jackets had been discarded and he wore the then regulation protective colouration: the dark grey suit and white shirt of the professional man. For the rest of his life, that was what he wore; he called the casual uniform of jeans and

*Memoir of a Thinking Radish, p. 118.

pullovers "fancy dress"—at any rate for himself. He was by now sure of his powers, socially easy and marvellously good-looking. He had become a good administrator as well as an experienced and brilliant research worker. I asked him once what he thought good administration was. He said, "It's what works."

I wondered a bit anxiously what it would be like to leave Oxford and live in Birmingham, an industrial town of about two million people, but I liked the idea of Peter being a professor at thirty-two, and began house-hunting. The Birmingham I visualised had smoking chimneys, grimy pale faces and a lot of bomb damage—this was only two years after the end of the Second World War. I need not have worried. Solly and his wife Joan had already picked out a house near them. Solly arranged for me to meet him at his home—far more elegant than anything we knew in Oxford.

Edgbaston, in the middle of Birmingham, turned out to be an oasis in which large comfortable houses sat in leafy gardens along tree-lined roads. The land is owned by the Calthorpe Estate and building on it was carefully controlled. The house we were to look at was built about 1760. It was called the Valley Farm, and was surrounded by an acre of garden. This garden was bounded by another big garden belonging to West House preparatory school for boys.

I knew at once that we should take the house. So we paid £2,500 for a ten-year lease and acquired five bedrooms, three bathrooms, and what the agent called three "public rooms," besides a cellar in which the earlier owners, so the agent said, had hidden from the violence of the Priestley rioters nearly two hundred years earlier.* The only snag about the house was the heating system. In the historic cellar was an inefficient boiler which Peter would have to stoke with solid fuel, and when I looked at the radiators I wasn't sure there were enough even to take the chill off

* Dr. Joseph Priestley's defence of the principles of the French Revolution roused a violent mob to attack his library and his laboratory.

the house. However, this snag was outweighed by all the other
advantages, and we began to plan the move from Oxford to Birmingham.

Peter went ahead of us and stayed with Dr. and Mrs. Rudolph
Peierls, where he enjoyed European cooking for the first time.
Caroline, now nine, stayed on in Oxford with the Professor of
Zoology and Mrs. Hardy to finish her term at the Dragon School.
Charles, aged five, and our *au pair* girls—Eivor from Sweden and
Irma from Switzerland—travelled in the movers' van; and I drove
with three-year-old Loulie in the very fully loaded car. The moving men, their load and the children arrived after a journey they
had all enjoyed, but so late that the men had to camp out in one of
the bedrooms. They got the furniture sorted out next morning, and
by the time they left the atmosphere was more like a picnic than a
move.

Gradually we settled into the new life. Peter could drive to the
University and his laboratory within ten minutes, Charles went to
West House School next door, and Caroline and Loulie could
easily walk together to their junior and nursery school round the
corner.

Peter was in peak form at thirty-three, and I never remember
his being tired or ill, except for a tendency to skin allergies. Someone once commented that this was a suitable nuisance for an im-
munologist.

The big garden was a joy. A shrubbery of rhododendrons sheltered a large lawn and on fine Sundays Peter organised games on
it. He and Charles loved cricket, so we played complicated games
of catch, either with a ball or a rubber ring. Peter would act as
though he had no intention of throwing the ball to any of us and
then in a second he had it whizzing to whoever least expected it.
He and Charles vied with each other at throwing the ring high into
the air and being the first to catch it, and he and I competed at
fielding catches, just higher than my arms could reach. I had to

jump, while he just seemed to reach up without effort.

In the summer holidays we were invited by Mr. Field, the headmaster of West House, the school next door, to use their swimming bath. Charles got a good basic education at this school, and he and Caroline and Loulie learnt to swim well. Mr. Field was a splendid man with a sense of schoolboy humour. On one swimming sports occasion, drenched by rain, to the delight of the parents he set an example to the boys by jumping into the pool with an umbrella over his head.

During the war, when gardeners were called up for military service, the big Edgbaston gardens had become wild—wild enough for foxes to trot in from the countryside to make their dens in the undergrowth and to pick up an easy living from dustbins and chicken coops. In part of the garden an area of rough grass was fenced off, and here Charles tried raising twelve baby chickens, bought in the market, hoping to augment his pocket money by selling eggs. The chicks that weren't eaten by foxes all turned out to be cockerels, so his first business venture wasn't a success, but we did eat the last one, accepting that the foxes would if we didn't. Unfortunately, as neither Peter nor I fancied wringing its neck, it had a flavour of laboratory ether.

In our third year in Birmingham, Solly Zuckerman decided to resuscitate the Lunar Society—in the form of broadcast discussions between various scholarly people. The original Lunar Society had been founded in the middle of the eighteenth century, before the days of electricity, so its proceedings had been arranged to coincide with evenings when the moon was full enough to light the members to the meetings. It became the leading provincial scientific society (at a time when the influence of the Royal Society was slight), and no wonder, considering the membership: Josiah Wedgwood, Dr. William Withering, James Watt, Matthew Bolton, Joseph Priestley and Erasmus Darwin. The ideals of the French Revolution, the possibilities opened up by the invention of the steam engine, the discovery of oxygen, all unleashed spectacular visions, and it was not surprising that Wordsworth had written, "Bliss was it in that dawn to be alive." In those days there was great hope of progress in the air.

The so-called Lunar Society of the Air broadcast some six unscripted discussions between—amongst others—Professor (later Sir) A. J. Ayer, Noel Annan (later Lord), Patrick Blackett (later Lord), Charles Madge, Sir Julian Huxley and Peter, not all speaking at once but in different combinations and on various topics. One discussion on extra-sensory perception caused a lot of interest. The modern participants were just as talented as their predecessors, but because of broadcasting, their ideas went further afield.

In our first winter the house felt cold and I had a stove put into the nursery; this also had to be stoked, by opening two doors in its front surface. These doors had little panes of mica through which you could see the fire either glowing, or sulking, whereupon you would open a lever to increase the draught. One late afternoon I thought I smelt singeing coming from the nursery. I ran in and found Charles placidly reading, with his back against the mica doors. When I turned him around, eight small brown squares were scorched into the grey flannel jacket of his school suit. In 1948 everybody still had clothes coupons and a school suit needed a good many, so I had to cannibalise pieces from an old jacket before he could wear it again.

By now our two *au pair* girls, Eivor and Irma, had become part of the family. (When Eivor, the Swedish one, visited us again in 1983, she was hardly changed except for the addition of a seventeen-year-old daughter.) So Peter was domestically well looked after—apart from duties with the coal-eater in the cellar—and he began to undertake an enormously energetic programme of lecturing, demonstrating, research and reading.

He was now in a position to help people younger than himself, and whenever he could, he did. Sometimes he steered a young graduate in a direction different from the one he had chosen—always to advantage. He helped his students—he referred to them as his "little chickens"—to prepare their scientific papers properly, or write their grant applications correctly, both of which tasks he did superbly well.

In Birmingham I can't ever remember going out with friends to a restaurant—I don't think there were any good ones—and what there was of theatre, opera and orchestras was limited. There may have been groups of friends who entertained each other in various ways, but we didn't find them, perhaps because we were there for less than four years; or perhaps Peter may have appeared too alarmingly clever to invite home. At the time, with three children and one to come in 1949, two *au pair* girls learning English and teaching me recipes, Peter's huge programme of work, and many visitors, neither of us missed not having many like-minded friends. We did go to concerts given by the City of Birmingham Orchestra, and when the competitive cooing of the roosting pigeons didn't ruin the pianissimo passages, they were fine. The pictures in the Birmingham Art Gallery and the Barber Institute were also a great pleasure.

Peter took his duties as professor very seriously, though he was himself more interested in physiology and experimental biology than in traditional classification and anatomy. Besides teaching his share of the curriculum, he soon became involved in experiments prompted by meeting Dr. Hugh Donald on a trip he had made to New Zealand in 1948. Dr. Donald had asked him if he could suggest a foolproof method of distinguishing between fraternal and identical cattle twins. Peter claimed that he had confidently replied, "My dear fellow, in principle the solution is extremely easy: first exchange skin grafts between the twins and see how long they last. If they last indefinitely, you can be sure they are identical twins, but if they are thrown off, you can classify them with equal certainty as fraternal twins." So when Dr. Donald wrote to ask if he would demonstrate the technique of skin grafting to a veterinary research team based at Cold Norton, an experimental farm forty miles outside Birmingham, Peter felt morally obliged to comply.

Accordingly he and Rupert "Bill" Billingham, who had come with him from Oxford, travelled to the farm and began demonstrating how to take a small piece of skin from one calf and graft it onto another. The results were not at all what they expected. They were impossible to reconcile with what they knew about the natural history of skin grafts in all the other animals they had studied. The explanation of the results came, as Peter wrote in his *Memoir of a Thinking Radish* (1986), "not through any exertion of our own but from reading the work of an American geneticist, Ray D. Owen, described in a book called *The Production of Antibodies* by Frank Macfarlane Burnet and Frank Fenner." As cattle twins share a placenta, through which the mother nourishes the embryo, the twins are literally transfused with each other's blood during development and each treats the other's as if it were their own. This explains why the power to reject each other's grafts was absent; it had been subverted before birth. Peter and Bill Billingham published their findings of the phenomenon, which they called "tolerance," in the journal *Heredity* (Vols. V and VI of 1951 and 1952).

Peter was often late back from the grafting experiments in the cattle shed at Cold Norton Farm. On one occasion I was beginning to be worried when the telephone rang. It was Peter, explaining in a rather thick voice that he had been in an accident, that the car was a write-off and a few of his back teeth had been dislodged. When he was driven home and I saw the state of his face, I was glad the children had not seen him come in. I was expecting a baby in a few weeks and wondered if it might be shocked into arriving early, but he wasn't. Ten days later, on 7 February, also my birthday, a second son, Alexander, took so long in appearing in the labour ward of the Queen Elizabeth Hospital that I had time to solve a *Times* crossword clue Peter and I had been puzzling over. When I thought of the answer, I sent word to Peter in his laboratory—partly to show off and partly to reassure him.

That year—1949—was a good one to remember. We celebrated Alexander's and my birthday, our twelfth wedding anniversary, and Peter's thirty-fourth birthday together, at home with the family. Then came another cause for celebration: the news that Peter had been elected a Fellow of the Royal Society. It was Royal because it had been founded by King Charles II in 1660. Fellowship, especially at a young age, confers an instant accolade which every scientist envies or respects.

Later that year Peter was visited by Dr. Gerard Pomerat, who was travelling on behalf of the Rockefeller Foundation of New York as a sort of talent scout, offering financial help to scientists thought worth backing. He put it to Peter that it might benefit him academically to spend some little time in America.

Peter described his reaction to this suggestion on page 116 of *Memoir of a Thinking Radish:*

I told him it would be a very great thrill for me to spend a few months sitting at the feet of Peyton Rous in the Rockefeller Institute, at the time the foremost centre of biomedical research in the world, and in many respects the model of institutions such as the National Institute for Medical Research in London.

I explained to Dr. Pomerat that as a salaried servant of the University I couldn't simply get up and go, and that I ought in any event to confine my visit to a matter of three months or so, a period during which I should be able to accept an invitation from Harvard University to deliver the so called Prather Lectures to the assembled biologists. Pomerat approved of my plans and said that the Foundation would make it possible for me to visit a whole number of centres in the United States and make contact with scientists I particularly wanted to meet.

When everything had been efficiently arranged by the Rockefeller Foundation, Peter sailed for America in September 1949, on the *Mauretania*. He didn't think the crossing came up to those he had made to South America on the Canadian Pacific liners in the twenties, but it gave him some relaxation and he enjoyed the gambling—and winning—in the ship's casino.

The day after landing he went to call on his patron, the Rockefeller Foundation, at 49 West 49th Street in Manhattan. He had "formed a mental picture of an elegant little terrace of houses of which one, No. 49, would be marked by the complete lack of ostentation characteristic of the enormously wealthy." No. 49 turned out to be the tallest building he had ever seen, one of the skyscrapers that make up the breath-taking ensemble of Rockefeller Center, and the office was on the fifty-fifth floor. He wrote me that his hosts could not have been kinder or more solicitous for his welfare and that they had handed him "hundreds of dollars" for his travels and expenses.

He was introduced to Dr. Peyton Rous and found him not only charming and kind but a man of enormous culture, learning and scientific achievement. In the lunch room of the Rockefeller Institute, Dr. Rous introduced him to a galaxy of scientists whose names were household words to scientists. Peter was fizzing with stories he wanted to tell about homografts and twin cattle and was invited to many a laboratory where he told them and exchanged ideas, as was his favourite occupation.

He enjoyed giving the Prather Lectures at Harvard, the first he had given in America. He spoke to the audience instead of reading from a paper: he had an exciting story to tell and told it with clarity. From then on he received a stream of invitations to visit or lecture in other universities or laboratories.

During this visit to New York Peter was given so much hospitality, and when he wasn't ate so cheaply at an automat called Bicks, that he amassed enough dollars to bring me over for a holiday. I travelled on the *Queen Mary,* second class, but the bursar promoted me to a shared first-class cabin, with real beds. I fell out of mine in a storm, quite relaxed, and happy to be on my way to join Peter. He was waiting at the dockside, full of plans to show me all he had learnt about New York. In front of the Rockefeller skyscraper he told me to look up. The top floors were in the clouds and I had to bend so far back to see the summit that my American grandmother's sealskin hat fell off into the snow. The luxury of the things in the shops, the kindness of the friends Peter had made, the rich food and the glories of the Frick and the Metropolitan museums made an intoxicating change from the austerities of post-war England. It was also a joy to see Peter through American eyes. They appreciated him with genuine warmth and with the sort of openness that in England would be found embarrassing. I loved it and didn't find it embarrassing at all.

When we came back to Birmingham, life was much quieter, though not for Peter because he found to his dismay that in his absence he had been elected as Dean of Science. This job involved much that he disliked—ex officio chairman of all committees, election to Chairs, and the need to have a thorough understanding of all faculty business. He said he regarded being Dean as an "intolerable distraction," particularly when he had to present all the science degree candidates to the Chancellor of the University, Anthony Eden. He was no good at pronouncing foreign languages, so I was impressed by the pains he took to master the names of the overseas students, and they appreciated it too.

The relatively even tenor of this life was briefly interrupted only a week after we got back from America. Peter was reading in the sitting room and I was mending, when we heard a sound like sizzling bacon. As I opened the door of the sitting room to see if there was anything going on in the kitchen, I was met by a blast of hot air from the open door across the hall, followed by smoke and a few crackling flames. Without a word Peter raced upstairs to get the sleeping children down and into the garden, and I dialled the Fire Service. A slow voice asked disinterestedly: "What sort of fire is it?" I remember saying crossly, "It's burning my back."

Anyway, the fire brigade arrived quite soon and found the flames coming from a cupboard in which I had stored paint pots, tennis rackets and newspapers; nobody had noticed two unearthed wires at the back of the cupboard, ready to spark and ignite the contents. The firemen couldn't help doing a good deal of damage, but the room needed decorating anyway, and the neighbours and children enjoyed the excitement. Before the firemen came, we made a chain of buckets to the pond in the garden. We had to stop when the children begged us to be careful of the goldfish and it became too dark to see what was drawn up.

In the summer of 1951 when Caroline was thirteen, Büdi brought a French family to visit us, to see if Caroline and their daughter of the same age would like to exchange holidays. Büdi had perhaps exaggerated Peter's academic standing, so the family had dressed themselves to impress. As they stood in the entrance hall, seven-year-old Loulie appeared, in her nightie and barefoot, at the top of the stairs, holding a small bottle and a glass. Without any embarrassment she slowly descended and offered it to the father of the family, M. Walberg, saying, "Would you like some *deadly poison?*" In spite of this Caroline was invited and the exchange was successful.

After almost four years in Birmingham, an alternative to the intolerable distraction of being Dean arrived. Peter received an offer to submit his name as a candidate for the Jodrell Chair of Zoology at University College London—the longest established of all chairs of Zoology in England. Rupert Billingham—Bill—was willing to move to London, and Leslie Brent, ex-president of the Students' Union and a very bright scientist, had become immensely keen to join in the research Peter and Bill were doing on the material obtained from the cattle twin experiment. So Peter applied and was elected, and we prepared for our new life in London.

SIX

Life in London, 1951

THERE WAS NO Solly Zuckerman in London to choose
a house for us, and house agents' descriptions of
suitable homes were so misleading that house-hunting trips based on them were a waste of time. I learnt
to ignore adjectives such as "immaculate," "spacious" and "luxurious." In those days chests of drawers were lined with newspapers, not the special elegant paper now available. One day, as I
tidied a drawer and folded a sheet of an out-of-date *Times* to the
right size, an advertisement leapt into focus. It was for a Queen
Anne period house and garden in Hampstead, freehold, for £15,000.
I immediately took the train to London—a two-hour trip—and on
the same day arranged to buy Lawn House, Hampstead Square,
for £10,000. It had been on the market long enough for the owner
to be glad to reduce the price for a quick sale.

Lawn House was on four floors, three for us and the fourth for our mothers—Peter's mother in the summer months and mine in the winter. Peter had never asked for a study, and I never thought of it, so one end of every sitting room we ever had was always lined with bookshelves and there Peter concentrated on whatever he was reading or writing, regardless of the noise from the nursery or elsewhere. I once asked him, in a mock interview, "To what do you attribute your concentration, Dr. Medawar?" "Application," he said, and when I asked what style he aimed at while writing, he answered, "Clarity."

To raise enough money for the new house we sold our car and did without one for a year. Peter travelled to University College on the Underground line. Sometimes on fine mornings we walked over a part of Hampstead Heath which led to the bus stop. He started thinking about his work, in spite of the amazingly rural and beautiful 880 acres of the Heath, almost as soon as we started walking. He was patient with my repeated requests to "just *look* at that, Peter," and gave whatever it was a quick approving look. When he looked as if he were really thinking, at home, I learned to ask, before interrupting, "Are you thinking?" and if he was, I didn't start talking.

At this time he smoked a pack of cigarettes a day—a habit I disliked, but I never remember him smelling of cigarettes. I do remember watching how the smoke from his cigarette drifted towards his reading lamp through the white silk lampshade I had just made. So I was thankful that when the first report on the correlation between smoking and lung cancer was published in 1950, Peter gave up smoking. This wasn't easy, and after a week or two he was restless and a bit irritable. I threatened that if this went on, I would have to start smoking, to calm *my* nerves. I bought him a substitute for nicotine called "Lobelline," after the Dr. de l'Obel who discovered the flowers called lobelias. It was supposed to be harmless and not habit-forming. Although Peter stopped smoking completely and claimed that he consequently felt much fitter, he often thought, even after a few years, how much pleasure a cigarette would still give him.

His resolve was strengthened when he was later on appointed Director of the Institute for Medical Research. "I could, in this job," he said, "perhaps justify rape, murder, barratry and arson—but not smoking, not after Doll's evidence."

One of the first things Peter did on becoming Jodrell Professor at University College was to arrange two rooms for the use of his predecessor, Professor D. M. S. Watson and his secretary. He also kept a room for distinguished visitors from overseas—"visiting firemen," he called them—that was in turn occupied by Paul Russell, Jerry Lawrence and Paul Terasaki, all American medical men come to learn about the immune system.

Peter greatly enjoyed his colleagues' company in the Department of Zoology, especially at tea-time. David Newth, Richard Freeman, Mary Freeman, John Maynard Smith, J. B. S. Haldane and his wife Helen Spurway, Anne McLaren, Alex Comfort and Donald Michie provided conversation which, he told me, was the best and most amusing he had ever heard or even expected to hear. The premises, however, did not match the people. The rooms were small, the windows grubby, the passages long and cold, and Peter's salary was inexplicably below the top of the professorial scale; but the atmosphere was stimulating and "matey," a quality Peter held to be essential for fruitful research. No time was ever wasted in rivalry or intrigue. The names of the authors of the papers published were always arranged alphabetically, instead of according to precedence.

Members of the department often slipped out of the dusty premises for a pint of beer over lunch at the nearby public house, the Marlborough Arms, and conversation continued there as it did at tea-time in the laboratory. When there were guests, the beer in the pub was accompanied by large plates of fish and chips. Sir Macfarlane Burnet was treated to such a plate on one of his visits, and when he had eaten every chip, one of the group asked what he would now like for his meat course. Sir Mac did not recognise the schoolboy teasing, but Peter loved the joke and told it many times over, without any malice.

The game of bar-billiards formed part of the pleasures of the lunch hour at the Marlborough Arms. Peter's own arms—which he called ape-like—gave him a good advantage at the game. On one occasion, playing with David Newth, John Maynard Smith, Richard and Mary Freeman, he missed a shot he had extravagantly and manifestly proposed to win. He made a terrible grimace and pretended to break the cue over his knee. Unfortunately, he succeeded, and for a memorable second the scene might have come straight out of a Marx Brothers film.

At about this time Peter's appearance, with some of the staff, on scientific television programmes brought in a large crop of would-be students. He and his colleagues tried inventing questions which would elicit whether or not the candidates were intelligent, stuffed with facts, or were merely fascinated by the professor and his staff. One such question was "Why have you chosen University College for your degree?" They expected at least some shy reference to the qualities of the teachers, but none came. Instead, the most memorable reply was "Because it is within easy reach of all the four main-line stations."

Peter's time at University College was the most fruitful of his academic life; he ran a research programme, taught, served on the Agricultural Research Committee and University Grants Committee, wrote papers of great importance, administered the department and raised funds for it. Thanks to consistent support from America he had little difficulty in raising money for his own research, but to raise money for his colleagues' research—for example, into the behaviour of spiders—he had sometimes to apply for money to nineteen different sources.

In the summer the great relaxation was playing village cricket. Of the departmental team, Leslie Brent was the only real sportsman, having played hockey for the combined English universities. Leslie roped in staff, female as well as male, graduate students and visiting Americans, most of whom became devoted to the slow, unfamiliar, ballet-like game, played at weekends, mostly on village greens, sometimes even in sunshine, always accompanied by pints of beer at lunch and home-made sandwiches at tea-time.

Squash was a favourite winter game, but one winter a craze for chess swept through the department. Peter told me that, at its peak, every time he wanted to visit one of his colleagues and put his head round the door to see if they were busy, they were, deeply pondering their next move on the chess board.

This was the period of the Supermice—the mice who demonstrated the phenomenon of immunological tolerance. Peter, Leslie Brent and Rupert Billingham worked intensively to "bring about by design the immunological phenomenon that occurs naturally in twin cattle, namely, to reduce, even abolish, their power to recognise and destroy genetically foreign tissue."* In order to reproduce in mice the situation they had observed in the cattle twins, unborn mice had to be exposed to "foreign" cells early enough in life for them to be fooled, as it were, into accepting such cells as "self" and part of their own make-up.

In the experiment they designed, a small dose of skin cells from a white mouse was delicately injected into each mouse embryo, easily visible through the body wall of its brown-furred mother. There was a lot of trial and error before they found the right dose of these foreign, "non-self" cells and the right stage of development at which the mouse embryo would accept them. The mouse family lived in a big, round, sawdust-carpeted glass container, covered with a perforated zinc lid, through which the stem of their

Memoir of a Thinking Radish, p. 132.

water bottle reached down to the right height for the mice to suck drops out of it. Finally a family of brown Supermice was born, and as each developed its coat of brown fur, it was grafted with a patch of white skin, from the white mouse which had provided the shot of foreign cells before it was born. The mice accepted the graft as part of "self" quite specifically: they were still able to reject a graft from a different strain of mouse.

This family of mice was lively and bright; they soon learnt that if they stood on their hind legs and all pushed up together, they could dislodge the lid. They dislodged it before anyone noticed. One of them sprang out, dashed across the room and disappeared down a hole made by an ill-fitting gas pipe in the floorboards. Unfortunately this space was the home of a wild house mouse, and the battle for territory between them was fierce enough for the squeaks and scuffles to be heard above. Everything was tried to induce Supermouse to return—a pretty female mouse in a oneway cage was placed just beside the hole, cheese, Puffed Wheat and milk was offered. Nothing worked, and when a defeated Supermouse finally crawled up through the pipe hole, his fur was bedraggled, his ear torn and he had lost much of his body weight. He was cossetted like a head of state, but the experience had been too much for him, and he died a sort of hero's death still bearing the graft of white fur. The survivors provided material for the paper in *Nature* in 1953 on what Billingham, Brent and Medawar termed "immunological tolerance."

The experiment of the Supermice was a brilliant success, one that established beyond all doubt the phenomenon of immunological tolerance. The discovery was particularly valuable in the field of surgery. Surgeons and scientists could now begin searching for harmless ways of suppressing the body's ability to reject grafts of much needed skin or kidneys.

Mice had always played a large role in the Medawar family. Peter modestly acknowledged that any fame he had achieved had been made possible by "climbing onto the shoulders" of mice. When we were living in Oxford, the children kept a family of very tame and extremely elegant black and white mice. These mice took a lot of their exercise running up and down each child. Strains of pure-bred black mice are very fastidious in their habits. After a journey from one laboratory to another, they refused food until they had spitted, combed and polished themselves all over, and remade their beds of fine wood shavings.

Peter had the idea of inventing a family of alphabetical mice. We were delighted whenever we thought of a new member, but we stuck at thirteen. We thought this was enough to make a book if only we could find an illustrator who understood and liked mice as much as we did. We admired Giacometti's drawings of Max the hamster, and hoped he might also like to draw mice, but unfortunately he didn't warm to mice as much as we did, though he liked the idea.* Here are the thirteen characters:

A = Anonymous
B = Bigamous and Blasphemous
D = Dormouse
E = Enormous
F = Famous
I = Infamous
L = Lachrymous
M = Magnanimous (this was the character Peter liked best)
P = Polygamous, Pusillanimous, Pseudonymous, and Posthumous (how on earth could he be illustrated?)

In London, Peter's scientific colleagues from Europe or America were always "passing through," the children's friends came in and out, and Peter was enormously busy. For anyone with a comfortable income and good health, London was a glorious place to be entertained in—by concerts, operas, theatres and cinemas. At

---

*After the war was over we wrote to him in Switzerland to ask if we might call, and we did.

this period too I could forget to take the key out of the front-door lock, without fearing the worst when I got home and found it still there.

I bought my first diary in 1953, and it makes extremely dull reading—just times of dental appointments, who is coming to stay or to dinner, which child had mumps, when to be ready for circus, school play or opera—nothing like a journal for a record of feelings. Peter never kept anything but his desk diary, in the lab, and that was perfectly looked after by whoever looked after him.

In London Peter could indulge his taste for opera. Several specialist shops sold out-of-date records and on Saturdays he often visited them to add to his collection. One desk drawer soon filled up with the programmes of operas we went to at Covent Garden or at the Coliseum, and another drawer filled with theatre programmes. The range of what we chose wasn't wide, but the volume was large; mostly we went to any opera by Verdi, Wagner, Strauss or Puccini. Wagner and Puccini are full of moments of tragedy or glory, guaranteed to move Peter to tears, and sometimes to sobs. He joked about it: one day, he said, a member of the St. John or Red Cross Ambulance Brigade on duty would at last find something to do, would put a hand on his shoulder and escort him from the premises. Mozart, Rossini, Strauss and Mussorgsky did not tap the tears, and so for me these were naturally a little more enjoyable. Our taste in plays agreed: Shakespeare, Ibsen (if we were feeling strong), Congreve, and Oscar Wilde gave such marvellous pleasure that we tended to be unadventurous about other playwrights.

A regular foursome played bridge nearly every week: Peter, his mother, sister Pamela and her first husband Sir David Hunt. They loved the game, played for only a little money, and wrangled and joked at the time and afterwards. I didn't feel out of it because I hadn't started, as I knew I was no good at cards.

Our youngest child, Alexander, was six in 1955 and at a morning nursery school just round the corner from our house. We had the same good strain of *au pair* girls, started by our Swedish friend Fritiof Kogge in 1946, to help with the household. Peter was now well known as a scientist and as a writer; he was in demand for lectures and committees and became more and more pressed for time. Besides membership of the Agricultural Research Council and the University Grants Committee, he served on the committee of the Runnymede Trust, founded to monitor the state of race relations and to improve them whenever a chance arose. One day I heard a story about Peter from Tom Rose, and from Dipak Nandy, both members of this committee. While Peter and they were members, there had been accusations of harassment of Pakistani families by the police in the borough of Ealing. The police did not co-operate in Runnymede's investigations of the story. Sir Robert Mark, Chief Commissioner of the Police, was asked to meet the Runnymede members in the house of Sir Jock Colville, then the chairman of the committee. Towards the end of the meeting Sir Robert turned to Peter, who had so far not spoken, and said, "Sir Peter, I am surprised that you, a man of science, should lend your name to anything so unscientific as this so-called research." Peter replied quietly, "Sir Robert, it ill becomes you, who know the value of evidence, to criticise Runnymede's work when your force refused to co-operate in this enquiry." He elaborated on this point, and when he finished Sir Robert was silent.

Around this time a desire to learn more came upon me; Peter's talents were Olympian and mine were largely domestic. I felt like stretching. I tried—and probably tried too hard and earnestly—to be both mother and father, to make up for the time he couldn't give to fatherhood. I went to evening classes in Russian and prepared to take an exam at "O" level (the point at which sixteen-year-olds take it), and I translated a book by G. V. Lopashov on the development of the vertebrate eye. I made the effort because I was moved by a naïve hope of influencing the Russian visitors to

Peter's lab. If only I could talk to them in Russian they might understand the folly of fearing the West, and so on. I had had the same dream about Hitler during the war. I dreamt I would meet him and get him to see that there was no such thing as race, only the human race. In the dream, Hitler's ambitions were mollified and he even appeared glad that we had talked, thus saving him and his country all the ghastly business of war. What actually happened was that when Peter's Russian visitors heard my fluent greeting they were fairly overcome with joy. Eyes filled with tears, they embraced me and answered with a torrent of Russian which I couldn't understand.

It was a childish idea, but at least it led me to the pleasure of translating Lopashov's book. I could not have managed all the details of its embryology without a lot of help from David Newth, who had by then left the Zoology Lab to become Professor of Medical Biology in the Middlesex Hospital Medical School. After a year I could enjoy Chekhov's play *The Cherry Orchard* in Russian, performed in London by the Moscow Arts Company.

In December 1955 the Soviet Academy of Sciences invited Peter to lecture at the University of Moscow. His views on the uniqueness of the individual, on Lamarckism, and on old age and natural death had not gone unnoticed.* I was included in the invitation and we both wanted to go; but in those days, the great Russian geneticist N. I. Vavilov had been killed in prison in 1945 and genetics was now in disgrace, and the views of the quack called T. D. Lysenko were in the ascendant. In Lysenko's opinion, all people were born equal, and how they turned out depended solely on their environment—an opinion which tallied usefully with the views of Russia's rulers at the time.

How could Peter be sure that his lecture would be truthfully translated? Might what he said be twisted to match political re-

---

*Published by Methuen in 1957 as a book, *The Uniqueness of the Individual*.

quirements? We debated a lot before Peter decided that if he were a scientist, living in a country which did not allow scientific independence, it would inspirit him to meet and talk with someone from the outside; so we went.

The first thing I remember about Moscow is the feeling of ice-cold air going up my nose. It was so cold that I thought the fluid in my eyes would freeze. We were quickly met, bundled through Customs—where I noticed the officials smiled in a friendly way—and into a large black car. We drove sedately into Moscow. Everything looked grey or black, or white where the snow had not been touched. As we reached the suburbs we saw formless women, swaddled against the cold, wielding shovels to keep the December streets clear of snow.

The hotel was large, warm and old-fashioned—especially the unpolished brass bathroom taps, encrusted with verdigris. We were shepherded around by Mikhail, a pleasant interpreter, who shortly developed a bad toothache. I suggested that he should take a day off and go to the dentist. No, he said, the pain there would be worse than what he was suffering. When I said surely he didn't mind the prick of an injection, he told us that their doctors held such injections to be bad for the system. At that time, local anaesthetics were in short supply.

After a few days Peter asked Mikhail where Professor Vavilov was. Mikhail did not know. Peter asked about Lysenko. Mikhail had obviously not been briefed, but the next day he came back with the official answer. Peter interpreted the rather vague reply to me as "Lysenko—him plenty heap good man." This galled Peter, and he scoffed to Mikhail about Lysenko's views as vigorously as was consistent with the manners of a guest. A year later Lysenko's star began to sink, but he was not discredited until 1964.

Our visit to the zoology laboratories was like a visit to friends. Their English was quite good enough to allow conversation to flow. In the evening they arranged a supper party, with dancing afterwards to a wind-up gramophone. There weren't enough men to go round but it didn't matter—I was whirled around by the ladies in Viennese waltzes while Peter sat out talking with the professor.

Tickets were bought for us to see Prokofiev's ballet, *Romeo and Juliet,* at the Bolshoi Theatre. Everything about it was superb. It was as though all the colour and design absent in the modern buildings had been reserved for the production of the ballet. We were used to marvelling at Margot Fonteyn's dancing. I thought no dancer would come near her, but Ulanova as Juliet was incomparable. She was then forty or near it, but as she ran barefoot across the stage with a scarlet cloak streaming behind her, she looked like a wild-eyed fourteen-year-old, desperate to reach her father confessor and get him to marry her to Romeo. Her movements were utterly beautiful—she raised the hair on my head.

Peter's lecture on immunological tolerance was held in a huge auditorium. They told us that eight hundred people had packed in to hear him. As he spoke, each sentence was translated on the spot, so the lecture took a long time. Some of the audience may have come to hear good English, but whatever they came for, they were enthusiastic and applauded with clapping and stamping.

As soon as the lights went out for slides to be shown, the Professor of Entomology sitting next to me—whom I had noticed, because he had rather long hair and very long nails—began to question me in a cautious whisper, in French, about life in England.

Peter often joked that there was no sleep so refreshing as that induced by the voice of a lecturer in the dark, and claimed that it was one of the greatest blessings that lay in his power to bestow. What with whispering back in French, keeping an ear cocked to listen how Peter was getting on, and recovering from nightly toasts of friendship-between-our-great-countries, I became so sleepy that I kept on falling sideways onto the professor, in a sudden relaxation of attention. He bore no ill-will, and when we left he presented us with a small case of butterflies, huge peacock blue ones from the eastern borders of Russia and samples of species from the different habitats in the vast expanses between there and Moscow.

Our last formal visit was to Professor General Pavlovsky. The professor was in a general's uniform and was not interested in us, except as objects to impress. He was very deaf and rather vain, and all we had to do was listen and look absorbed. As we got up to go, he signalled to the interpreter that he wished to give us a present. It sounded as if it was going to be a good one, and my spirits rose—perhaps it was caviar—but it turned out to be three plaster busts of himself, one for us and two to be delivered to admirers in England. We had to buy a suitcase in order to carry them, but there wasn't anything else to spend our roubles on, anyway. General Pavlovsky was such a perfect stage general that we enjoyed our time with him as if it had been a theatrical sketch.

Peter and I were moved by our Russian visit. In 1955 we did not know what was going on in the Gulags. Amongst the people we met, there still seemed to be an unspoken pride in Russia and in the original ideals of the Revolution. The Russians had survived the Nazi onslaught and they were untainted by the commercial pressures of the West. I had brought a copy of *Housewife*—the magazine for women at home in those days. After a week in Moscow I threw it into the wastepaper basket just as Mikhail came into the room. He noticed where it was and asked if he could look at it; as he turned the pages and saw the advertisements for brassieres and scent, "guaranteed to attract any man," I felt ashamed and wished I had brought something better.

But Peter could not have been a better representative of English scientific and cultural values. Until we were at home again, I didn't realise how much the Russian visit had influenced me. In England, in my generation, you got credit for running a good home, looking after your husband and keeping yourself in shape. In Russia this wasn't enough; they wanted to know what your profession was, and how good you were at it. I think this was one of the reasons why I began to work in a family planning clinic in Islington and in the Citizens Advice Bureau in Hampstead; in both I learnt how many people spent their lives in a state of quiet despair.

After a year at this work Josephine Clifford Smith, the general secretary of the Family Planning Association, invited me to take on public relations for the head office. There I began the great friendship of my life with its chairman, Margaret Pyke, and with her physician son, David. She was my ideal of a perfect mother and friend, and she had more influence on me than any woman I have ever met.

Her manner was serene, but lively and ready to be amused. All her qualities worked in harmony, so that she managed an even tenor of life in spite of considerable difficulties. Her father was a doctor and her husband the eccentric genius and inventor Geoffrey Pyke. During the war Lord Mountbatten co-opted him onto his staff, where he welcomed original thinkers. Geoffrey Pyke discovered, amongst other things, that a mixture of sawdust and super-cooled ice bonded together to make a rock-hard substance known as Pykrete—which floated in sea water. He was working on Operation Habbakuk to build fuelling and rest stations made of Pykrete in mid-Atlantic when the end of the war put a stop to this ingenious plan.

Margaret and Geoffrey Pyke separated in 1929, and Margaret was left with her young son David to bring up. She took a job as the secretary of Hayes Court School until Lady Denman appointed her as general secretary of the newly formed National Birth Control Council. Lady Denman was the powerful and much respected chairman of this council, and of the Women's Land Army. During the war Margaret moved into Trudy Denman's home, Balcombe Place in Sussex, and became her close friend and right hand.

I was first introduced to Margaret in 1954 at the headquarters of the Family Planning Association in Sloane Street, London, where she had become chairman on Lady Denman's death. Josephine Clifford Smith presented me as a new volunteer who was good at recruiting people to the cause of family planning. I felt instantly at home with Margaret. She was slight but quite strong, had silvery grey hair, observant grey-blue eyes and a beautifully shaped face. As she talked to me, I felt that she was not only interested in the public relations work I was doing for a birth control clinic in a rather seedy part of London, but that she was confident that I could become good at it. My education had not been strong on this sort of encouragement and it was just what I needed. I wanted to please her in the way a good child hopes to please its mother.

Before long I became a member of the executive body of the Family Planning Association and Margaret arranged that I should represent the Association at European conferences on family life.

Because I had four children, and spoke quite good French and German, I seemed to reassure the militant Roman Catholics who believed that anyone who supported birth control must be a hard case who didn't want or like children. The delegates at conferences on "The Family" often forgot my name, but the second time we met it was "Ah, my dear, I remember you—Mrs. Family Planning." Margaret then suggested that I should help her devoted son David to write and produce the quarterly journal he had started in 1952, *Family Planning*. He and his family had recently moved from Oxford to London, to Kings College Hospital, where he had been appointed as consultant physician, and this left him little time for the whole business of producing the journal, from commissioning articles to page proofs and editorials. So I started. I had to start at the top, as joint editor, because I couldn't start at the bottom; there was no office boy or girl or career structure to follow.

I loved it. David was a good teacher and with his encouragement I found that I had absorbed enough of Peter's writing to be able to edit long-winded articles into crisper ones. David asked me to review a book on the life of Havelock Ellis. I had never reviewed before and I took this assignment very seriously, even to reading Ellis's three volumes on human sexual behaviour. The review turned out all right and I was pleased that François Lafitte, Havelock Ellis's stepson, later told me that I had really understood his stepfather's life.

Peter was now covering scientific, literary and administrative ground at a ferocious speed, as well as flying around to give lectures in America and Europe. He never wasted time: he "accomplished the business of the day within the day," as the Duke of Wellington snapped at a lady when she asked how he managed to write longhand despatches from Spain as well as plan, fight, and win the battles against the French.

He answered letters in twenty-four hours and read each only once through, to save time; he laid out tomorrow's clothes before going to bed, never relaxed before a meal with a glass of wine, ate too fast and didn't sleep well. I once teased him into promising that he would not work on one evening a week and that we should have a proper two weeks' holiday every year. His defence against my protests about overwork was always a big smile and the assurance that he was different—he didn't need rests because a lot of his work was "as good as a rest." He achieved so much, and so much enjoyed achieving, that slowing down held no attractions. He was not able to sleep late, even on Sunday mornings when I found it difficult to wake up. Then, around nine, he would appear at the bedside with a slice of bread and honey and a large cup of what he called wake-you-uppo-tea.

When I became busy he gave me a typewriter, and when parking meters came in, a boxful of coins to feed them; but he wasn't good at giving regular birthday or Christmas presents, because finding the right thing takes a lot of time. So he asked me to go out and buy whatever I would like. "I expect you'd like me to wrap it up," I said, and he would laugh and say, "And don't forget to write on the tag: 'To my darling wife from her devoted husband.' " Perhaps I shouldn't have played this game. It might have been better for Peter's health to have had to do some easy, ordinary chores, but I got pleasure from thinking I was saving him for Higher Things and he constantly appreciated what I saved him. Later on, his present-giving talents enlarged. "I want to load you with jewels," he used to say, and once I let him.

Lawn House was pleasant for parties of fifty or so. At one of these, for members of the Society of Experimental Biology, a member of the Zoology Lab told me that he and some friends had agreed that Peter was a man who had everything; I had a primitive feeling that it was as well not to say this out loud. Somebody added, "He's good at everything except relaxing."

By 1957 Peter had written enough lectures on evolution, old age and natural death, scientific method, Lamarckism, tradition and immunology to make up the book called *The Uniqueness of the Individual*. He wrote in my copy: "To darling Jeanie, our first book, from her loving Peter." The "our" was generous because my contribution had been limited to enabling, listening and sometimes simplifying. He typed it himself, mostly in the evenings with his two fingers, working as fast as a good touch typist could. At intervals he shouted with laughter as an idea amused him, and it wasn't the sort of brilliancy that occurs in the middle of the night and is a ghost by morning; that laugh always signalled a winner.

When Peter had first started writing in Oxford, some of his sentences were so long that by the end I had forgotten the beginning, and I complained. He soon wrote with great clarity, impetus and wit, very much as he spoke. Although he read comics as a boy, *Rainbow* and *Beano,* I don't think he ever read rubbish. After digesting Arthur Mee's *Children's Encyclopaedia* there were, for him, too many interesting alternatives: Russell, Whitehead, Thackeray, Trollope, Dickens or George Eliot. He regretted being unable to share my enthusiasm for Tolstoy, because, he said, "There are too many names per person." We became addicts of Jane Austen in 1938. In those days when you stayed two weeks in hospital after having a baby, I took in lots of books, *Pride and Prejudice* among them. When Peter came to visit, I was so absorbed by Elizabeth's unexpected encounter with Mr. Darcy in the grounds of his estate that I could hardly put the book down. I gave it to him soon after and he became just as admiring and absorbed as I had been.

The year 1957 was a good one for medals—first from the City of Paris and then from the University of Liège where Professor Fritz Albert, a remarkable surgeon, had become deeply interested in Peter's work on transplantation. The ceremony at which Peter received his honorary doctorate and medal was much more moving than most because there were trumpeters in the gallery above the hall who blew a fanfare, which lifted the proceedings above the usual ritual of solemn procession and catalogue of intoned names. The menus in Belgium were also more memorable than most and much more filling.

By the time Peter became a professor at University College in London he was offered many attractive and generous invitations to America; in March 1958, he accepted one in New York to lecture and meet colleagues. The children and I set off a few days later, before it was light, to drive to Cornwall for an Easter holiday. After driving 280 miles in ten and a half hours we arrived to camp in a caravan and two tents on the Roseland peninsula at Trewince Farm. There was no motorway then, and we had to drive at an average of about 30 miles an hour because we were trailing a 14-foot sailing dinghy behind us. On this holiday Loulie made friends with the sons of the farmer and enjoyed a lot of rough riding. I began to learn how to sail a dinghy. I wanted to make sure that we all knew what to do if we capsized, so I arranged an artificial sinking in one of the creeks of the River Fal where the

water was only just out of our depth. It wasn't, in those circumstances, as alarming as I had imagined. I took the bung out of the
floorboards and the water began flooding up into the boat. Gradually the sail smacked the water and then lay quiet in it. We had to
climb up onto the gunwale above the water level, let down the sail,
and then let our counterweight bring the boat upright. Later, I
often thought that the image of Sinking the Boat helped in facing
any sort of hazard—you consider what is the worst that can happen
and what you can do if it does happen.

Alexander, then nine years old, wasn't keen on sailing. The
first time we keeled over while sailing in a fine breeze, he curled
up in the bottom of the boat with his hands over his ears; he wasn't
keen on the heavy jobs either, like hauling the boat up out of the
water. Jack, the owner of the boathouse at Percuil, used to tease
him for laziness and call him Marmaduke, a term of abuse in the
local sailing club. However, years later Alexander made up for his
unseaman-like behaviour by sailing across the Atlantic in a small
ketch with a girl who couldn't sail but she could cook—and when
they landed after twenty-eight days, each of them could both cook
and sail. He didn't marry this splendid girl, but found another,
Avis, whom he married in September 1985 on the island of Nan-
tucket, with his brother Charles as witness.

When Peter returned from America to join us, his high spirits
were infectious. On long drives on the way to a new picnic place
he invented a game in which he, driving through a quiet village,
pulled grotesque and alarming faces whenever anyone looked at
us in the car. My role was to smile and appear totally unconcerned.
"They'll date their lives by that spectacle," Peter said, wrongly
assuming that village life lacked drama, but the children probably
gave the game away by the way they rolled about laughing and
encouraging him.

On the beach he invented the game of Roo stones—named for
Caroline's pet name, derived from Ca-roo-line. It was simple but

fun. A small tower of stones was built about 20 feet away and each player accumulated a pile of ammunition and tried to knock the top stone off. We scored only vaguely, but the competition was just fierce enough to keep us warm after swimming in the very cold Cornish sea.

One of the best beaches we ever found could be reached by only two routes: by sailing into it from round the arm of the headland; or by walking along the cliff top and finding a way down through sloe bushes and bracken to where an old rope dangled down, almost as far as the sand. This small beach had a large cave and sand martins built their nests in the cliff above. They wheeled about in great sweeping arcs twittering as they flew, paying no attention to us, even when we tumbled dead pine trunks over the cliff to make a glorious fire in front of the cave. We often stayed with a picnic until the tide came in and the waves rushed over the glowing logs; then for a second before their colour faded you could see their crimson shapes rolling gently about under clear water.

Early in 1959 Peter was invited to give the six Reith Lectures on "The Future of Man." These are the grandest of the British Broadcasting Corporation lectures and were instituted by a former Governor, Lord Reith. Peter read a small roomful of books on genetics, evolution and history, and spent many, many hours writing and condensing them. In his introduction to the book which the lectures became, he noted that "I should not myself have been so arrogant as to choose 'The Future of Man' as a title for these lectures; but I am glad now that it was proposed to me, because it made me think more widely than I had done before; and this, I believe was part of the British Broadcasting Corporation's intention when it founded the Reith Lectureship."

He gave the first lecture on Sunday 15 November 1959. He began by explaining that the lectures were to be about the process of foretelling and would not foretell anything. Anyone who hoped that he was going to pontificate on Man's Future was disappointed.

What he talked about in this lecture was the fallibility of prediction, which he illustrated mainly with the problems raised by trying to predict or regulate the size of a human population. It was a dense, meaty and important lecture, appreciated by people who already knew a little of what he was discussing. Towards the end he said, "I should not be in the least surprised if in the 1970s or 1980s we in Great Britain were to start exchanging uneasy glances about the dangers of overpopulation, and wondering how things were going to end." He guessed rightly.

The last lecture on "The Future of Man" ended like this:

"The inference we can draw from an analytic study of the differences between ourselves and other animals is surely this: that the bells which toll for mankind are—most of them anyway—like the bells on Alpine cattle; they are attached to our own necks, and it must be our fault if they do not make a cheerful and harmonious sound."

The publication of the Reith Lectures again increased the number of attractive invitations to lecture abroad. Professor Barrigozzi of the Institute of Genetics in Milan invited Peter to give a lecture, in terms which he had taken the trouble to discover were likely to be accepted—two plane tickets and two seats for La Scala opera house. Unfortunately, the opera was not by Verdi, as we had hoped. It was Humperdinck's *Hansel and Gretel;* but we couldn't grumble—the music is pretty and there are no moments of glory or tragedy, so Peter got through dry-eyed. On this trip we were able to dine in Verdi's favourite restaurant, Savini's. When we had finished trout, Cervello al burro nero, pineapple with maraschino, and drunk Verdi's health, Peter sat back, smiled and said, "Let's have this at home." He enormously enjoyed this sort of free treat. He worked because he wanted to, but the rewards of recognition were sweet and he found it easy to enjoy the luxuries of life, especially when freely provided.

Next, Harvard invited him to give the Dunham Lectures in the early spring of 1960; the cheque that went with the invitation made it possible for Caroline, now twenty-two, to come with us. We stopped in New York and went to the Frick Museum, probably every visitor's favourite. Mr. Frick had lived in the style Peter said he would enjoy today. The pool in the middle of the house was not warm and chlorinated, but purely decorative; it was enclosed by arched cloisters and banked with sweet-smelling white narcissi, planted near enough the edge to be reflected in the water. On the walls of the beautifully furnished large rooms were Rembrandts, Titians, Renoirs and Chardins. What Peter wanted, he said, was a room large enough for him to invite me, after supper, "to take a turn" in it, as the heroes did in Jane Austen's novels. The Frick Museum gave him his first pleasure in looking at paintings; the way he ran his life didn't allow many opportunities, but it was a start. A few years later, when we were looking at one of Rembrandt's portraits of himself as an old man in Kenwood House, Hampstead, I noticed that Peter was moved to tears. Kenwood was another house he would have liked to live in—it had space, elegance, a well-furnished library.

After spending two days in New York, we left for Boston where we were welcomed at the Dana Palmer House, Harvard University's house for guests. It was well furnished with antique furniture and comfortable for sleeping, but there were no meals. For breakfast we walked over to the Faculty Club, where we were enrolled as visiting members. Breakfast was arranged on a self-help system and the atmosphere was very quiet. We sat at long refectory tables and opposite us, instead of talking heads, were rows of open newspapers. Caroline and I kept our voices low, but they couldn't help being English and audible. After a few minutes the newspaper opposite us was lowered. Behind it was a thin friendly face, with white hair and blue eyes. "Good morning," the gentleman said, "My name is Washington Platt." Then he smiled. "I have every reason to dislike the English—but I can't." He had been a brigadier general in the U.S. Army and had had some bad experiences with his opposite numbers in France. He belonged to the Sherlock Holmes Society and was planning a trip to England next year to visit the famous house at 221B Baker Street. We became friends: he helped us to feel at home and he promised to visit us in Hampstead when he made his trip to London.

Of all the hundreds of lectures, from many clever people, that I have ever listened to, these three Dunham Lectures were the best constructed and most brilliantly delivered that I have ever heard. In them Peter presented the whole story of immunological tolerance and its implications. He wanted people to understand what he was talking about, and he had taken pains to be understandable. He had timed each hour's written-out talk to the minute, condensed the lecture into notes with key words as reminders, and spoke directly to the audience. He did not stay behind the lectern but walked up and down as he spoke, as though supercharged and unable to stand still. At his request, the lectures were not published. His view was that, once published, he could get, as he said, "no further mileage" from them; he wanted to be free to deliver them, refreshed and augmented, on some other occasion. The Dunham Lectureship Committee's report on the lectures noted that "Dr. Medawar had been an exceptionally satisfactory lecturer, in terms of the originality of his work, its significance for many areas of biology and medicine, and the graciousness which characterized his period of residency."

Whilst Peter visited laboratories and met colleagues, Caroline and I were shown the sights by Dr. Guido Majno and his wife Fritzi. He treated us in a manner to which we were not accustomed, presenting one of us with a white and the other with a dark orchid; he took us to the Tea Wharf, the Cordova Museum and the studio of the sculptor Mirko, and generally looked after us while Peter was busy. This began a friendship which has grown over twenty-eight years.

After Boston, Peter went south to New York and Caroline and
I flew to Montreal to stay with Mrs. Lindsay, the mother of Jeffrey
Lindsay, one of the Canadian bomber pilots who had lived with us
in Oxford while on leave during the war. We had never met, but
Mrs. Lindsay was a legendary figure to the children because of the
food parcels she had posted to us from 1943 onwards, packed with
delicious things from Canada. Staying with her was like going
back to my childhood. The house was large and comfortable and
was maintained, from below stairs, by old retainers, while Mrs.
Lindsay organised charities upstairs, remembered the birthdays of
her six children and their children, gave elegant lunch and tea
parties, and smocked dresses for the grandchildren—as good as
those for sale in the most expensive shops. It was very cold while
we were in Canada and I wondered how the ladies stood the up
draught of icy winds in the street. I learnt how they did it at one of
the lunch parties when they went upstairs to the bedroom to take
off their coats. As each coat came off the outer skirts were flipped
up, without unnecessary modesty, and thick, long-legged woollen
bloomers were pulled off and laid on the bed beside the coats.

It was spring when we got back to London and Peter began his
normal round of teaching, research and conferences. Alexander,
now eleven, went back to his day school in Hampstead, and I to
my evening Russian lessons. Charles, a strong young man of
eighteen, went off to the *Theta* sailing club in Norfolk; Caroline
(twenty-two) went back to Cambridge University, to prepare for
her final degree in English; and Loulie, who left school at sixteen,
went by train to Grenoble to study French for an advanced level
examination.

That summer Peter had a lot of writing to do and a huge research
programme to finish, so he joined us in Cornwall for only a short
break. For part of this holiday the caravan at the farm was let, so
we camped in a field on level grass above a tidal creek. Twice a
day a family of swans sailed down the tide for their breakfast, and

home again in the evening, catching their supper on the way.

Early one morning I woke to the sound of snorting and trampling. A herd of bullocks had found their way through a gap in the hedge into our field and were coming at a trot towards the tent to investigate. I was frightened that their hooves would tangle in the guy ropes of the tent and that it and they would collapse on top of us. Luckily I was scared enough to remember a vision of Mrs. Barbara Woodhouse (who understood how to communicate with dogs, horses and cattle) blowing down her nostrils, as she quietly introduced herself to an unbroken horse. I stuck my head out of the tent and blew down my nostrils, murmuring shakily in what I hoped was a soothing voice, "Would you mind getting the hell out of here." After a few bellows and what I interpreted as looks of astonishment, the herd withdrew.

We stayed on after Peter left, but I promised we would get back home by 7:00 p.m. on 29 August, and we did. He came out of the house to the garage when he heard us arrive. He looked very ill, and was in great pain, feverish, and his face and neck were alarmingly swollen. He had neglected a bad toothache—because he wanted to finish a run of experiments before we got home; the toothache had got worse, he had the tooth out, started on penicillin and reacted very badly. I helped him into bed and rang our doctor. She came, gave him an injection of antihistamine, and within a few hours the fever and swelling went down. But Peter didn't feel well for several days. Later that week we were invited to the opera *Aniara*. He didn't enjoy it and felt bad enough to leave before the end—most unusual for him.

I felt anxious about the next undertaking: driving a new car across Europe to Prague. Peter had been invited by Dr. Milan Hasek to speak at a meeting in September, arranged in a hotel in the Tatra Mountains in Czechoslovakia. Milan had constructed Siamese chick twins while each was still in its own egg; just like the cattle twins, they accepted skin grafts from each other when they were fledged. I felt less anxious when Dr. Jean Deinhardt, a devoted graduate student of Peter's, and her doctor husband Fritz came from America to stay with us, and decided to accompany us as far as Hamburg. At Osnabrück, the Deinhardts collected a Carman-Ghia car which they had ordered from America. They were expected at the factory, and we arrived on time. All the papers and the car were ready—it had even been run in, on the bench. We drove the cars in convoy to Hamburg and stayed there in a beautiful hotel on the river. After we left the Deinhardts I did a lot of the driving as Peter was still not feeling quite well, and we drove on to pick up Charles who was staying with a family at Ratzeburg, in order to learn German. He was very glad to see us, especially because he had spent the last two weeks hoeing turnips and said he hadn't learnt any good German at all.

For the next leg of the journey to Vienna, Charles sat beside Peter and they took it in turns to drive—Charles had got his driving license that summer. From the back seat on the first day I watched with anxiety as a small spot swelled up on the back of Peter's neck; his allergy to penicillin had not quite subsided. I was relieved when we reached Vienna. There we were met and looked after by the Corcoran family, friends of Charles's. The swelling went down without treatment during the next two days and Peter began to feel better. We celebrated his recovery by dining in a restaurant called the White Chimney Sweep and afterwards went to see two old Charlie Chaplin films. Charles laughed so much and so helplessly that the people in the seats around us laughed as much at him as at Charlie.

I had tried to get visas for Prague in London. The atmosphere in the Czech Embassy there had been chilly, unsmiling and un-helpful; the most help I could get was advice to obtain the visas from the Czech offices in Vienna. We accordingly made our way there and joined a dreary queue of people waiting to get visas to enter Czechoslovakia. Round the room were openings in the wall where clerks sat, protected by wire mesh and a vertical sliding shutter which they could slam down to end a conversation.

When our turn came, I got nowhere. I insisted on seeing a higher official; we were taken behind the shutters to explain our needs to a surly superintendent. He told us that it was impossible to give us visas—either we should have got them in London, or we must wait some weeks in Vienna while he filled in forms in triplicate. I felt a sudden cold fury, and as we had little to lose, I told him in German that my esteemed and distinguished husband had been invited by the authority of the Czech government and the president of the University, and that of course, if we could not enter his country, it was of no importance to us, but it would be to our hosts, who would hold him entirely responsible for our absence.

To our surprise, he disappeared with our passports and after a while came back with our visas. When we returned to the waiting room, our success and relief must have shown because several people begged us desperately for help. They had been waiting for days and hoped we might have influence or advice that they might use. All we could do was commiserate. Next day we left Vienna regretfully, without time to explore, and drove on towards Czechoslovakia.

When we reached the frontier, Peter noticed that it was guarded with a high wire fence and that the barbed wire and the top was arranged to slope inwards and down, not to prevent people entering the country but to keep those inside from leaving it. The frontier guards were not the sort to exchange pleasantries with and they searched the car sullenly, as though they were looking for stolen goods and would be pleased to find them.

The atmosphere changed when we found the hotel in Prague— there a delighted Milan Hasek was waiting to welcome us. After a good dinner and a long sleep we felt better about his country. Next morning he drove us to the airport and we were squeezed into a plane barely big enough to hold Peter, and flew northwards to the Tatra Mountains. As we circled to land, I saw that there was no runway—just a long dry field surrounded by beautiful mountains. The landing was bumpy but nothing broke. A car was waiting for us and we were driven to a rather grandiose hotel where the staff were waiters and cooks in training, fresh-faced, and eager to please. The next few days were spent in discussing the latest results from experiments of common interest with Milan and his colleagues and in glorious walks on mountain tracks.

After dinner on the last day, Milan collected a supply of bottles on a table amongst the palm trees in the hall and the group of immunologists settled round Peter; all of them were eager to meet him and hear him talk informally. As usual, he delivered beautifully. He always spoke clearly, and when talking to foreigners, he made a point of using the Latin form of a word instead of its Anglo-Saxon equivalent. The people he enjoyed meeting most were the young, who wanted to learn and had ideas they wanted to discuss. At intervals more bottles arrived and toasts were drunk "To England!" "To your country!" "To peace," "To friendship"—almost anything would do.

Peter was still not in his usual form, and from a reaction which the immunologists well understood, so he was allowed to say goodnight long before the Czechs' ideas of hospitality had been satisfied. I felt that the honour of England was at stake, ridiculous though it was to measure it by the ability of the liver to stand up to large doses of alcohol; I whispered to Charles that we must not be drunk under the table by our hosts. We managed to hold out, until affectionate goodnights were at last exchanged; by that time I was glad there was a bannister to hold onto as we climbed the stairs to bed. I got to the bathroom in time to be very sick, and I think Charles was too, so we did not feel hung-over next morning when we made the return journey to Prague for a party in Milan's house that evening.

We were dropped at a small hotel in the centre of the city. That evening Milan collected us from it in a small un-upholstered car. The light was fading as he turned sharply to the right off a main street and I heard Peter enquire, "What does that notice say?" What it said was "Danger, no entry—road up." I think Milan was over-tired. Next moment the front wheels hit something very hard and the car rebounded, only to crash the back wheels into something equally hard. The engine cut out, the car tilted to the right and we stopped where we were.

Where we were was over a six-foot trench in the road, with the left wheels balanced on a tramline that hadn't been taken up, and the right wheels resting on the granite paving blocks left over at the right end of the trench. Charles's upper canine tooth had cut right through his cheek, the right side of my face was beginning to bruise and swell, and Peter's face was running with blood from a cut on his forehead. I managed to get out and checked that the cut was not deep and that he was not knocked out. Obviously Milan was the most in need of succour—he was standing by the car in a state of shock and what he was thinking could not have been clearer if it had been written in a captioned balloon. "What have I done? I should have seen that notice. I may have damaged Peter's brain."

I hugged him and told him not to worry because I was sure we were all right. In no time we were surrounded by a ring of onlook-ers, some kindly handing out tablets of painkillers—how and why did they have them? An ambulance was sent for, and by the time it arrived one of the onlookers had fallen into the trench and was included, with difficulty, in the ambulance with us. At one point the ambulance man approached Peter with a first-aid kit and what I thought was a hypodermic. I was so scared that the contents might be penicillin that I biffed his arm up, shouting, "Penicillin nyet!" His face in the dusk expressed "another mad English-woman," but he didn't persist, and Peter was spared whatever was in the hypodermic.

The ambulance was like an ordinary van, and had no blankets. By this time Peter was shivering from shock—more probably from the way he had to be inserted into the small van than from the cut on his forehead. It was cold, and I covered him with my coat. In the hospital I was not allowed with him into the treatment room; this was just as well, as no local anaesthetic was available and the lady doctor who closed the cut with two stitches included a piece of Peter's hair within the closure. We behaved as we thought the British were expected to behave and said that *of course* we wanted to come to Milan's party that evening; but we looked battered and were glad when we could decently leave to go back to the hotel and get into bed.

At the frontier next day, nobody remarked on or offered sympathy for our obvious injuries. "They're not surprised," Peter said. "They just think we've been beaten up."

We drove slowly home. It was very hot and we stopped for a rest in a place called Pilsen. There, for the first time, I drank beer and liked it. When we got home, the car was all right but we felt we needed a holiday.

SEVEN

Nobel Laureate, 1960

THE NEXT THREE WEEKS were full and tiring, but on 20 October 1960 a piece of news reached us that improved our lives as though we had been transported to a better world. My old friend Marghanita Laski rang me in great excitement and began giving congratulations. When I asked her "What for?" she said, "Oh dear, haven't you heard? I don't think I should be the first to tell you." As I couldn't stand the suspense, she soon told me that Peter had won the Nobel Prize for Medicine—sharing it with Sir Macfarlane Burnet, who had been working along different lines on similar problems. Peter had already heard the news and had tried to ring me, but the University College telephone lines had become so loaded with incoming calls that he hadn't been able to get through.

There are several paintings of Danae, receiving Zeus in the

attractive form of a shower of gold; she looks surprised, stunned and enchanted, just how I felt when the news sank in. Peter immediately became a numero uno, a man who had received the ultimate scientific accolade—and as far as I know, everyone thought he deserved it and no one grudged him the reward. Apart from the honour and glory there was a cheque for £15,000 to spend as we liked.

Peter gave a large share to his mother, to his colleagues Leslie Brent and Rupert Billingham, we bought a good refrigerator and a large Bokhara rug. The man who sold it to me said, "If you are tired of it in ten years, bring it back and we'll be glad to buy it at the increased value." I could never get tired of it.

Invitations to the Nobel celebrations in Stockholm included the prizewinner's family, and accommodation in the Grand Hotel. Only Loulie was free to come, and having her with us made the fun greater for us. We set off in great excitement in new coats, with a new suit of tails (the second since 1937) for Peter and beautiful new evening dresses for Loulie and me. The expedition is pure pleasure for the family of a Nobel Prizewinner. Unlike the laureate, you have no responsibility to deliver the lecture of acceptance, or give thanks at the huge formal banquet, and so are free to enjoy the magnificent yet friendly hospitality.

We left for Stockholm in the comfort of first-class seats on the Swedish airline, and settled down to enjoy the champagne and Smorgås for a couple of hours.

As we were approaching Stockholm, the plane began to lurch and bump. The pilot informed us that we had run into a violent snowstorm and would probably not be able to land. Peter had closed his eyes and was clearly entering that stage of nausea when you hope nobody is going to speak to you or ask you to move. Loulie became as pale as ivory and was feeling very ill. I felt queasy, but Loulie's distress saved me from worse. I stroked her forehead and murmured soothing phrases about the storm being over soon; they may not have done her much good but they kept me busy and therefore from being sick.

At last we stopped circling and hoping to land in Stockholm and the pilot's voice told us that we were going to spend the night in Germany. This was an anticlimax, but once we were out of the storm we felt better, and after landing safely the whole thing became part of the new Nobel world. I don't even remember which town or hotel we were in—everything was done for us, so gracefully that it was easy to accept. We had no responsibilities, we were tired, we ate well and slept deeply. Next morning we were seen onto a fast train to Stockholm. European trains always took me back to the excitement of my first travel abroad to Germany in 1932. They smell different from English trains, they move differently, and the food and service is, or was, not only different but better. The comfortable carriages ride high above the rails so you do actually descend to the platform, while sliding your hand down a brass rail for security.

In Stockholm a reception committee with the formal, friendly manners of the Swedes was waiting for us, and we were exposed to the first of many press photographers. Everybody seemed relieved at our safe arrival and pleased that we were not upset by the night's detour. From the moment we arrived, everything was done with a dazzling, fresh, imaginative elegance. It was impossible to realise that the Swedish people and the Nobel Committee had been delivering this kind of fairy-tale celebration every year since Alfred Nobel founded the prize—we were made to feel that welcoming us and honouring Peter was the one thing that they had looked forward to all the year.

Our hotel suite was full of flowers and messages, from Fritiof Kogge's daughter Nanette and the lovely *au pair* girls who had learnt English with us ten years before. A car was provided driven by a pretty, friendly girl, ready to go wherever we wanted, and an aide briefed us on every detail of protocol; he was equipped to supply anything from white gloves to safety pins. When I went to buy Loulie a pair of boots, speaking just enough Swedish to ask for them, I found that I had not brought enough money. I only had to murmur, *"Min Mann är Nobel Pris Tagare,"* and there were cries of joy, general excitement and no problems about payment "until convenient."

The ceremony during which the King of Sweden presented the winners with their gold medals was organised with great elegance and dispatch. Everyone was in full evening dress and decorations; even the two official photographers wore tails. The Nobel Committee and the prizewinners sat on a platform. When their turn came, they were escorted to meet the King, standing just in front of the audience, and presented to him. When he had read the citation and handed over the medal, the recipient walked back to his seat to the sound of vigorous applause. I don't remember what the music was, except that it was spirited and everyone felt elated by the time the proceedings were over.

After the ceremonies the reception and dinner in the Palace were as splendid as they could be. Peter came in with the eldest of the three Princesses on his arm and I was partnered by the Minister of Foreign Affairs, Herr Undén. I had been warned that he was not fond of social occasions; at dinner I asked him about the number of dinners he had to attend and if he would perhaps rather be at home or not have to make conversation. He responded warmly to this solicitude and turned out to be an excellent partner, both at the dinner and dancing Viennese waltzes afterwards.

During one of the intervals, the wife of a very wealthy Swedish industrialist came up to Peter, and I couldn't help hearing what she said. She gazed up at his face and growled in a deep 1930s film voice, "Hello, lover boy!" She was neither young nor lovely and Peter was alarmed enough to signal for help. When I came over, she amiably invited both of us to have dinner at her house. She entertained us lavishly and draped me with presents from a large chest, pulling out of it silk stockings and a beautiful silk shawl; and she made no further advances on Peter. We enjoyed her wonderful collection of furniture, pictures and treasures. She was a good hostess and, as Peter said, "Being rich is a very endearing attribute."

He had not grown up surrounded by beautiful furniture, china and pictures, and until he was in his early thirties and became a professor he had neither the time nor the money to spend on them. I think his first taste of elegance came in 1949, from enjoying the Zuckermans' house in Edgbaston where everything was a pleasure to look at. There comfort, taste and inherited antiques were well combined, and his ideas of what he would like around him expanded considerably. After we bought Lawn House in Hampstead in 1953, we couldn't afford a car; but at the end of a year we were in funds again and Peter began taking notice of the way our house was furnished. At one breakfast he looked with distaste at the simple, wooden toast rack on the table and asked me to get something "better." I defended the toast rack and said, "Just the sort Wotan [the head God in Wagner's *Ring* cycle] might have had— and I thought you liked Wotan's taste." Well, he certainly liked his music, but I did buy him a silver expanding rack soon afterwards.

After the Nobel Prize we were Invited Everywhere, and we visited many beautiful houses and enjoyed them. Peter came back from Princess de Rethy's house in the Ardennes—where he was consulted about plans for furthering Belgian science—with admiration for her surroundings and hospitality. His bedroom, he told me, had, besides superb comfort, a cut-glass decanter of whisky beside the bed. Not in our house, I thought.

By 1962, when we left Lawn House and I was allowed to decide the layout and decoration of our new house, Peter took great interest in everything—we needed new curtains by this time, and before I bought the material to make them, I showed him patterns.

The aura of winning the Nobel Prize seems not to fade; from 1960 onwards Peter was deluged with requests to lecture, to endorse, to advise, to review, to join, sponsor or provide signed cabinet-sized photographs for autograph hunters. I wonder if there is—as there should be—an Association of Autograph Hunters. How much effort and disappointment the hunters could be saved if they realised that each signed cabinet-sized portrait they ask for would cost the sitter at least £10, apart from postage. Peter usually gave me the requests to deal with. We developed a code of practice in which curt demands without prepaid postage went into the wastepaper basket. Heart-felt, well-written pleas, with postage, got a signature but no large photo, only a note of its cost. If the writer seemed very young I sometimes wrote, rather priggishly, suggesting that the fame they sought would be more likely to come from their own efforts than from a collection of someone else's signature, however distinguished.

Besides autograph-hunting letters, a new sort of mail began to arrive. One American lady sent Peter a story in which she, in the form of a rather wet spirit, clothed in white, appeared to him at frequent intervals as his muse and guardian. She pictured him wearing tweeds, smoking a pipe and striding out moodily for lonely walks with his dog. He pencilled in the margin, "No tweeds, no pipe, no dog," and said, as he gave me the letter to deal with, "A clear case of mistaken identity." Public recognition reveals how many desperately lonely hearts there are in the world. The saddest letters were from people who had read accounts of his transplantation experiments and wrote begging him to use his skills to graft back a limb severed through some terrible accident.

One direct result of the prize was an invitation from a very remarkable Syrian, Emile Bustani. He had a deep and passionate love for his own country, Lebanon, and also for England. He had come to London for an operation and while recovering in St. Mark's Hospital he learnt that Peter's father had been born in the

Lebanon and had lived there as a boy. He immediately got in touch with Peter and invited us to stay with him at his home in Beirut.

Nothing could have more resembled a ride on a magic carpet. We were flown first class to Beirut in August 1961 and were welcomed on the airfield by Emile Bustani with an entourage that included photographers from his Commercial & Trading Company (CAT) and others from Lebanese newspapers. Peter was used to such attentions; I was not. By the end of a week in which our every move outside the Bustanis' house was photographed, I felt too exposed to move from it. Peter kindly did that day's engagements alone and I slept all day and recovered quickly.

Emile's hospitality was Eastern and sophisticated. He and his wife Laura knew how to enjoy themselves and how to share their pleasure with others. At one of the parties he gave in their beautiful house at Yerzeh, on the hills above Beirut, I saw how important it was for many of the very smart guests to be photographed shaking hands with Peter or even—second best—kissing mine. After an hour I extricated myself and went up onto the flat roof, just above where the party was being held. From there it was easy to see why the stream of people shaking Peter's hand had seemed endless: it was constantly augmented (like the circulating crowd in lavish productions of Verdi's *Aïda*) by people passing back into the house and returning for another handshake, in the hope of being more favourably photographed than in the first round.

Emile's love and admiration for England included a passion for Winston Churchill's speeches. He had a record of the one that encouraged England to fight the Nazi menace and hidden amplifiers to broadcast it round the garden. Towards the end of one of his parties, the familiar lisping voice spoke clearly out of the darkness between the trees: "We shall fight them on the beaches . . ." It may not have moved the party-goers but it moved us to swallow sudden tears.

The kindness of the Bustani family is unforgettable—we were

treated like long-lost family. They sent us everywhere on the magic carpet, to stay in the splendid St. Georges Hotel—now a bombed ruin—to visit Byblos with Professor Zeine Zeine, the most sympathetic and learned director of the museum at Byblos, to visit Jerusalem in one of Emile's private planes, and to Amman and the Dead Sea.

The tourist trade has spoilt so much of Jerusalem that though the visit was interesting, it was not at all moving. I had a dysentery-like attack which made a misery of the obligatory progress along the Via Dolorosa: I had to knock on the door of a convent and beg for urgent asylum.

The Dead Sea and Amman were much more fun. While floating in the sea, I splashed some of the corrosive salt water into my left eye. Peter bounced towards me, almost able to walk on the water, and licked my eye like a cow—the only possible treatment. Even then, the eye became quite sore and red. Later on that day we were invited to a wedding in Amman. The ceremony required a lady acolyte to dance round the altar, I think three times, throwing eau de Cologne over the kneeling congregation each time she circled. I lifted my head to see the dance and whispered to Peter, "Watch out, here she comes again." This was a reference to an old *New Yorker* cartoon by Geo. Price, in which poison ivy is chasing a scrawny, beak-nosed man round his cabin in the woods while his wife, equally beak-nosed, stands rigid with fright as she calls out the progress of the poison ivy. Peter got a bad attack of helpless giggles and I got an eyeful of eau de Cologne—serve me right— so I got a second red eye. The magic carpet arrangements flew us back to London on 6 September, glad to have been invited to Lebanon and yet glad to be home again.

The normal accumulation of letters waiting for us included an invitation from Professor Carlos Chagas in Rio de Janeiro. In exchange for one lecture, the University invited us as their guests for a week, with an honorarium besides the plane tickets. Peter's brother Philip was living somewhere "in the interior" of Brazil, looking for mica, and the prospect of seeing him and hearing his frequent helpless laughter, and perhaps even playing bridge with him, appealed to Peter.

A Brazilian admirer of Peter's wrote to tell us that after the announcement of the Nobel Prize, Peter had been billed in Brazilian newspapers as a "distinguished son of Brazil." Anyone born in Brazil, whatever the nationality of the parents, becomes a Brazilian with a Brazilian passport. So though Peter's mother was British and his father was naturalised British, he had both a British and a Brazilian passport. He had not fancied visiting his birthplace after he grew up because it might have put him at risk of being conscripted into the Brazilian Army, which would not have suited either him or it. We tactfully checked that no form of conscription was included in the invitation.

The travel arrangements for getting to Brazil were quite complicated: we were to start in Paris on 9 December, and from there would catch a Lufthansa plane going to Cologne, thence to Dakar on the coast of West Africa, and on across the South Atlantic to Rio.

The flight to Paris was simple but the Lufthansa plane to Cologne never arrived. We spent a noisy and uncomfortable night at a hotel in Orly Airport and left early next morning for Cologne. Hours and hours later we landed with a heavy bang at Dakar Airport—the impact had burst a tyre. I am always surprised that does not happen more often. We didn't get to Rio until Monday the 11th at dawn—about 5:50 a.m.

It was a strange entry. The car that met us at the airport drove very fast along a modern motorway towards Rio; at one point it swerved to avoid something lying in the fast lane—it was the body of a man. We realised he was dead because two lighted candles were burning beside him. In England the ambulance would have arrived to take his body to hospital or to the morgue, without considering where his soul might be going; but here the candles represented a fond hope for his afterlife.

Our hotel was on the Avenida Copacabana, facing the Atlantic. We unpacked, had breakfast, and, taking the risk of ending on the road with candles beside us, crossed over to the beach for a first swim. Bathing on Copacabana Beach was a great experience, as Peter taught me how to face the enormous incoming rollers. He had learnt as a boy that when a huge wave rolls towards you as you are standing up to your waist in sea water, you should put your hands together in front of your head and plunge into the wall of water. You emerge undrowned, and surprised to find yourself on the other side. During the visit we spent all our free time in the sea playing this game of porpoises.

Then, after the swim, we tried to sleep off the long journey. I was woken up by violent, enduring cramp in my left leg—not the sort that goes when you press your foot on the end of the bed, but the sort that makes footballers fall down on the pitch and twist about with the pain. Peter helped me to get to the bath and sprayed hot and cold water in turn from the shower, and the board-like muscles very gradually relaxed, perhaps because of his first aid. This was my first but not the last experience of bad cramp. Over the years I have been told of various cures; sufferers can choose between a raw potato in the bed, a cork held between the feet, quinine sulphate, and selenium extracted from yeast.

In the afternoon we pulled ourselves together and set off to visit Professor Chagas, Peter's host. He was the son of the man who had discovered the disease which bears his name, and he and Peter had corresponded about the possibilities that the disease Charles Darwin had suffered from intermittently all his adult life was Chagas's disease.

Peter believed that Darwin had been bitten by the Great Bug of the Pampas, the vector of the infection, when he landed in South America during the voyage of the *Beagle*—a view with which

Professor Chagas agreed. The alternative theory credits Darwin's symptoms to a psychological illness. As the evidence for the correctness of either theory cannot increase, their adherents are unlikely to change their views.

Peter gave his lecture in an ordinary lecture room, from which the windows opened onto the noisy Avenida Atlantica. There were not more than one hundred in the audience and they did not seem rivetted by what Peter said—there was a lot of rustling and scratching and looking out of the window.

One day our hosts took us to Petropolis where Peter had been born. I remembered his Mama telling me that the hospital had at that time been run by nuns and that the beds had no sheets, only rough blankets that harboured fleas. There were then no nurses— all the nursing had to be provided by relatives. We were not shown the hospital but were given a rather grand lunch instead and were glad of the choice.

During the week's visit I was asked what I would most like to see in Brazil. I said I would like to visit Brasilia, the city in the interior of the country where four rivers meet, and which had become the seat of government in 1960. A trip was arranged, the way these things are when you are a visiting foreigner. We flew there over forests and mountains and it was like landing in a new world: the light was intense and the air clear, dry and hot. Over the new city, which looked like a scene from the film *The Shape of Things to Come* based on H. G. Wells's book; the sky was immense, arched like a dome instead of the familiar transparent ceiling. Many of the public buildings for the ministries were tall and thin and, we were told, could be used only half at a time: in the morning the sun baked the east side too hot to work in, so the staff changed over into the west half; only after midday could they move back to their eastern quarters.

The President's Palace was beautiful, with arches for shade and a fountain playing in a wide pool by the entrance. Many of the other buildings were suffering from concrete "cancer" as we could see when we came close, but the general effect was imaginative and exciting.

The intellectual atmosphere in this city was quite different from Rio. There was an air of hope and excitement and energy, and the scientists showed real delight at meeting Peter. One man proudly showed his copy of one of Peter's books and even mentioned a reference to my thesis on lymphocytes. It was easier to be hopeful in the high air of Brasilia, away from the 80 million people concentrated in and around Rio, half of them illiterate and half of them under voting age. In Rio, the contrast between rich and poor was horrible; we were taken to visit one house where there were two swimming pools in the garden but only lean-to shacks with banana-leaf roofs at the gates for the servants. The drawing room in this house was cool white, except for the lemon yellow of the sofas and pale gold of the orchids flowering in pots around the room. When I admired them, the hostess immediately broke off a whole wand of flowers. Some of the chairs had seats of Aubusson tapestry. I asked what happened if they needed repair. The answer was simple. "They are sent back to Aubusson." I wish we could have met the Brazilian Archbishop Camara, who spoke out bravely about the social system. Four years after our visit he and several of the clerics denounced the government's apparent indifference to the vast inequalities in Brazilian society and became champions of the right of dissent.

The only shopping we did was when Peter bought me a small ring, which I somehow lost on the aeroplane. A few weeks after getting home, someone sent us a newspaper article about our visit; it was not about Peter's lecture or his visits to the medical school, but about how mean it was for a Nobel Prizewinner to buy only one ring when he had accepted an honorarium. They probably thought that we were very rich; but it would not have occurred to us to spend a lot of money on luxuries. Perhaps after all it was for the size of the prize that the invitation to the "son of Brazil" had been made.

At the end of the trip Peter went to visit Philip in a small town in the region of Govanador Valladares and I flew home by myself. It was so hot at the airport in Rio that the sweat ran down the faces of the black porters. On the plane I had a seat next to an elderly German who asked me what I had liked best about Rio. I said the lack of racial prejudice—how pleasant it was to see black, brown, white and all shades between, strolling and sunning and swimming on the beaches like members of the same species and not as if they were different "races." He gave me a lecture on the subject of race and how concentration camps had "only existed in the imagination of journalists." I felt too angry to speak. I stared coldly at him and rang to ask the stewardess for another seat. When we landed in Portugal the temperature was down to freezing. I was glad to get home to London and to a moderate climate.

EIGHT

Director of the
National Institute, 1962–1966

I
N 1962, PETER WAS INVITED to become Director of the
National Institute of Medical Research in Mill Hill, seven
miles from the centre of London. This Institute is the
largest of all those for which the Medical Research Council is responsible. He was delighted to be asked and was proud of
the appointment, and quite glad to exchange the grimy windows
of the Zoology Department for the splendid large view from the
Institute building, set in the green landscape on the border of
Hertfordshire.

A house went with the job. It was built late in the eighteenth
century, was surrounded by a walled garden and perched on top of
Mount Vernon, at almost the highest point of Hampstead Village.

I was invited to tea there by the retiring Director of the Institute,
Sir Charles Harington. Lady Harington poured out and I sat op-

posite her on an old sofa. I shivered with cold and shifted about to avoid a loose spring. The Haringtons lived austerely, did not notice the cold, and had not liked to ask the Medical Research Council for repairs or decorations all the time they lived there, so a lot needed to be done. I particularly noticed the bare boards in the only bathroom, wide enough apart to admit spiders, and the single swan-necked light fitting above the bath which would not have shed enough light to see even a large spider, should it emerge to scuttle under the bath.

After looking all over the house I told Peter that it would be just right for us if it could be made warm, and white and waterproof. This request caused endless difficulties in the administrative offices of the Treasury and Medical Research Council. When Peter's appointment had been made official, he had confirmed that we would like to move into Mount Vernon House and we promised to sell Lawn House to friends. We then waited so long for a date by which the restored house would be ready to move into that Peter became upset and frustrated—so upset that he carried a small radio round with him, to distract him from thinking about the situation.

We could make no plans for months. Peter's frustration was caused by a conflict between his gentlemanly manners, his intense dislike of rows (he once told me this came from a fear that he might boil over and regret it) and outrage at the position we had been put in. Finally, I warned that unless he did something to break the impasse, I would go on domestic strike. He was sufficiently alarmed to write a letter of dignified protest to the Council, notifying them that unless a decision about repairs to Mount Vernon could be rapidly reached, he would resign from the post of Director "in circumstances which would make it impossible for any honourable man to succeed me."

Arrangements were shortly made for the repairs to start. I suggested the addition of two more bathrooms; there would then be a small, self-contained flat on the top floor for our mothers, and another in the basement, each with their own front door, and another small flat on the first floor, in addition to the main rooms of the house. I was pleased with this idea, because when our turn came to leave Mount Vernon I thought it would make a fine house in which the Medical Research Council could instal visiting scientists—and the design was approved. But when we left in 1974, twelve years later, the house was turned into offices. I never went back inside after we left it, but from the outside I noticed that the golden climbing rose I had planted in 1963 which had reached the top of the fire escape had been cut to the ground. While we lived there we filled the house with four nearly adult children, our mothers in turn, a niece, a spare room for visitors, and an *au pair* girl. I had a good time planning details with the building department of the Medical Research Council, making curtains, getting our worn furniture repaired and floors covered. What the builders called "completion day" was 23 August, but we did not move into Mount Vernon House until November 1963.

The house was now warm and comfortable and everything about it pleased us. It had been cold, leaky and rather neglected; now it was in order, full of colour and comfort. It was right for us, yet flexibly arranged for whoever came after us.

When everything was finished, the house and garden looked beautiful. We decided to celebrate with a party. We invited the first Director of the Institute, Sir Henry Dale, the retiring Director, Sir Charles Harington, and every member of the staff who had been there in both Directors' day and was still employed there.

As Sir Henry Dale's ninetieth birthday was very near, I ordered a huge cake. We added an appropriate number of small candles and lit them as he came into the room. He arrived with a piece of sticking plaster on his forehead, apologising for being a little late; he explained that he had been delayed by falling downstairs, but now felt in good form, as he demonstrated by making a short welcoming speech.

Peter greatly enjoyed the responsibility of being the Director of the National Institute. Before he began and before we moved house, while the family and I were on holiday in Cornwall, he learnt the names, faces and work of the two hundred people in the Institute with the help of a book of photographs. Then he came down to Cornwall for a week's holiday. During that week he demonstrated how incompatible he and my 14-foot sailing dinghy—*Seal*—were. He was about half as tall as the mast and only just under half the length of the whole dinghy.

One morning he was standing nonchalantly on the small deck of *Seal* when one of the children ran down the stone steps cut in the harbour wall and jumped into the boat. As it lurched, Peter slipped and grabbed the mast. His weight, applied so high up, catapulted me from where I was standing by the tiller into the water of the harbour, to the delight of watching holiday makers and of course the children.

Peter began his time as Director of Mill Hill (the short name for the Institute) by arranging weekly lunches with the heads of the various divisions. He was lucky to inherit Sir Charles Harington's superb secretary, Pauline Townend, without whom he "could not have done," as he often said. In his travels, he observed that whenever a big institute or university ran particularly well, there was always a Pauline Townend at work, filtering back to the director aspects of administration he might not have thought of, and executing the actions that followed.

During Peter's time at the Institute, it became a Mecca for immunologists. The money to run the National Institute is supplied by the Medical Research Council—which in turn receives it from the Treasury. Peter once described the system as "same cow, different teats." Once in the coffers of the Institute, the Director is responsible for allocating the money to the different divisions. Then the head of the division—Cryobiology, Biochemistry, Animal Husbandry or whatever it may be—spends it as he thinks fit, but is responsible to the Director for the success or failure of his plans.

In any Institute, morale depends a great deal on the temperament of the Director, his relations with the Medical Research Council, his ability to attract research workers who achieve good results and his understanding of the progress or stagnation of each individual's experiments.

Apart from being a good Director, Peter's example of keeping up his research encouraged work in every department; he kept two and a half days a week clear for his own research and he made it his business to keep up with the progress of everybody's work. He put into a Director's Fund any earnings from television interviews made during office hours; and this money went to help members of the Institute to travel abroad to conferences. One of his innovations was the institution of a bar, to encourage a relaxed exchange of ideas, problems and solutions. Besides carrying on his research and giving lectures, during 1963, his second year as Director, Peter fitted in nine trips abroad and visited eight universities.

He ran his scientific life with great speed and efficiency and the efficiency was not bought at other people's expense. He knew that things mostly get done because people like each other, so he took care to consider the welfare and feelings of the members in his research team and of the Institute. As he wrote in 1979, "one of the benefactions of increasing age and experience is the realisation that everyone gets on better if a generally matey atmosphere prevails."* The atmosphere in the lab was not just matey—it was fun. In *Advice to a Young Scientist,* he also said that once a scientist experiences the exhilaration of discovery and the satisfaction of carrying through a really tricky experiment, then he is hooked, and "no other kind of life will do." It was marvellous luck, Peter thought, to be paid for an activity and way of life most of which

Advice to a Young Scientist (New York: Harper & Row, 1979), p. 58.

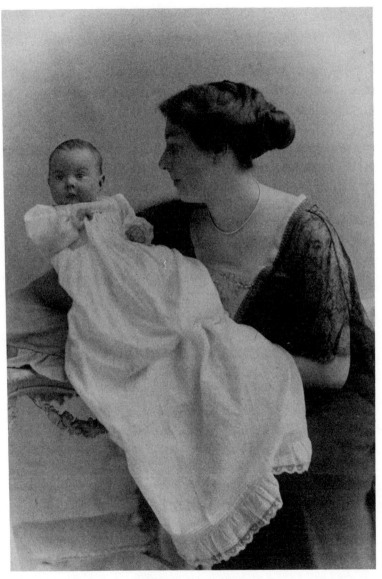

Jean Medawar and mother wore long dresses for this photograph, taken on May 18, 1913, to celebrate Jean's christening.

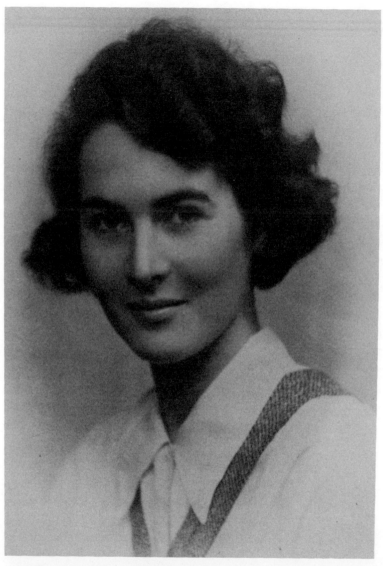

Jean was given a dress allowance at sixteen. "I spent most of it on a blue Harris tweed skirt held up by braces and made by a local Cambridge dressmaker."

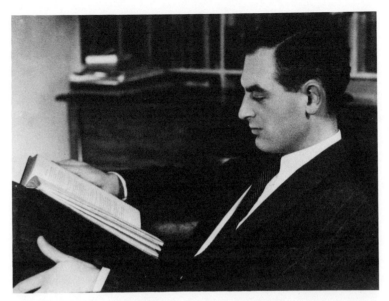

When Peter was twenty-two, the year we married, I persuaded him to have a formal photograph taken, at home in our flat, 110A Banbury Road, Oxford. He is relaxed because he forgot the camera while reading Sir Francis Bacon.

Tutors and pupils: The Experimental Biology Club, Oxford, 1946. Peter (second from right) was tutor to Avrion Mitchison (far right) and Francis Huxley (second from left), and was pupil of J. Z. Young, on his right. J. Z. Young is talking to the philosopher Karl Popper, who had an immense influence on Peter.

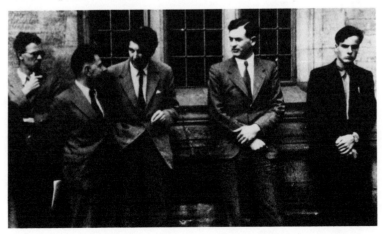

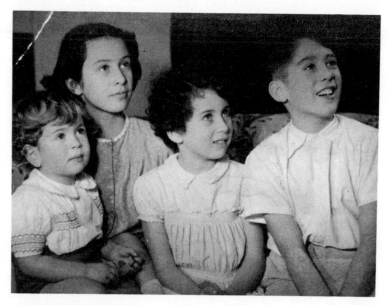

Our children in 1949. Alexander is on Caroline's lap; Loulie sits in front, beside Charles.

November 1960, in the sitting room of Lawn House, Hampstead, London. Peter is reading some of the telegrams of congratulation on winning the Noble Prize for Medicine, surrounded by (left to right) Loulie, me, Caroline, Charles (standing), and Alexander (sitting cross-legged). PLANET NEWS, LTD.

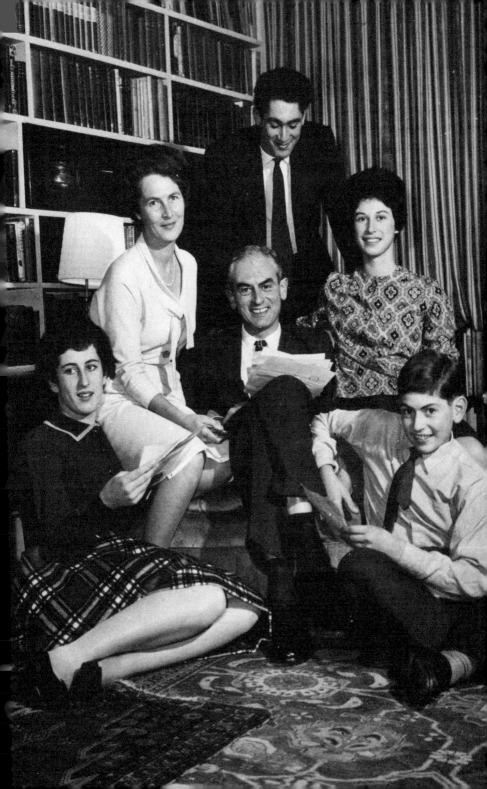

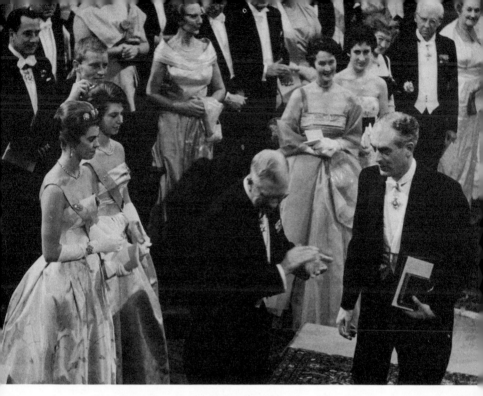

December 10, 1960. The Nobel Prize ceremony in Stockholm: (left to right) Princess Margareta, Princess Désirée, King Gustav of Sweden, me, Loulie, and Peter. AKE BORGLUND

Mount Vernon House, Hampstead, where we lived from 1963 to 1975.

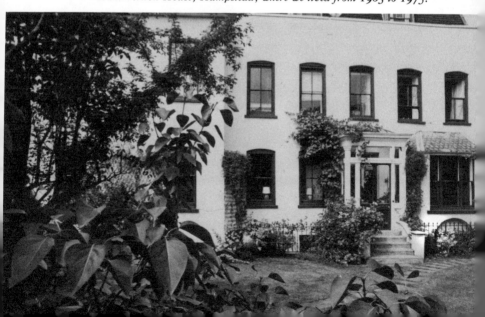

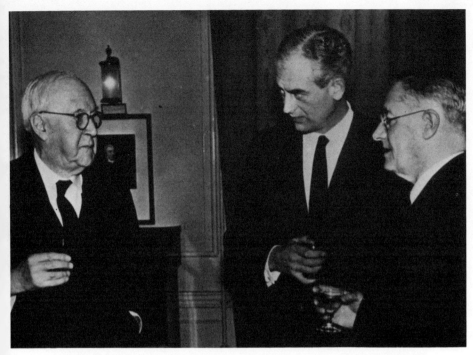

Three Nobel Prize winners, at a party given by the CIBA foundation to celebrate Peter's prize. Peter is talking to Sir Henry Dale, his predecessor at the National Institute for Medical Research, and Lord Florey, discoverer of penicillin, and his chief at Oxford.

1962: Director of the National Institute for Medical Research, London. UNIVERSAL PICTORIAL PRESS & AGENCY, LTD.

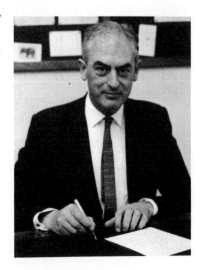

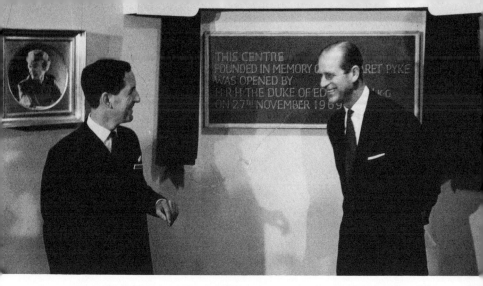

The opening of the Margaret Pyke Centre, November 27, 1969. Prince Philip unveils the plaque, watched by Dr. David Pyke. The picture on the wall behind him is of his mother, Margaret Pyke. CRISPIN EURICH

April 1970, on the beach in front of Victor Rothschild's house in Barbados, seven months after the stroke. Peter is trying to hold up his left half-paralyzed leg. Loulie came from Chicago to help us. Left to right: Benjamin, age five, Loulie's eldest child, and Siiri, age two.

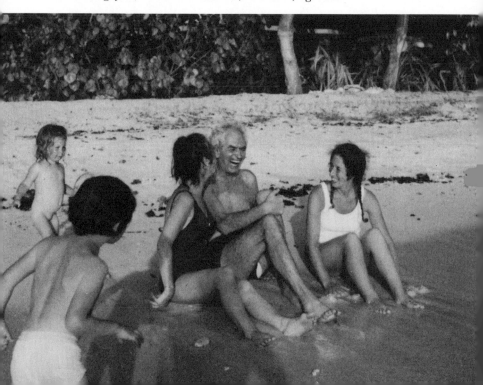

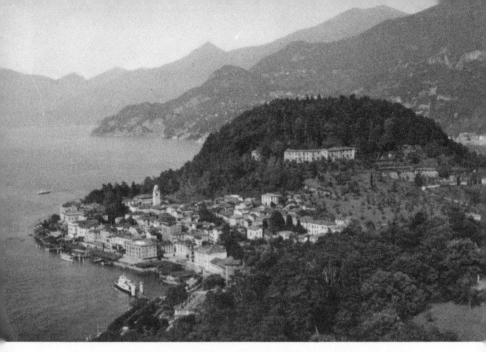

The big house in the trees halfway up the hill is the Rockefeller University's Villa Serbelloni, at Bellagio on Lake Como. Peter was a scholar in residence there in September 1972, writing From Aristotle to Zoos.

Outside the front door of the Villa Serbelloni, Peter is saying goodbye to Jacques Monod. Edna Healey is in the middle of the picture and June Goodfield in the doorway.

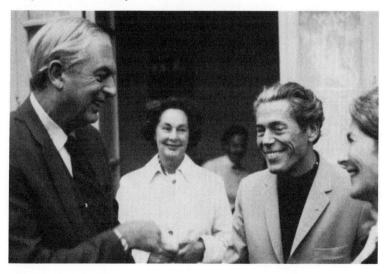

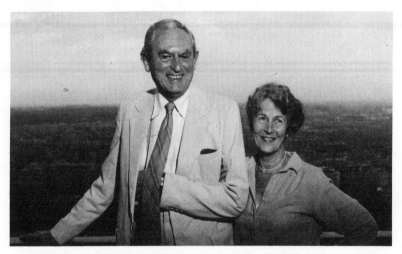

September 1978, on the balcony of the Hilton Cavalieri Hotel in Rome, at the International Conference of Transplant Surgeons. ELI FRIEDMAN

David Pyke was a faithful friend. Here, he and Peter are discussing the best way of refilling the pencil with one hand.

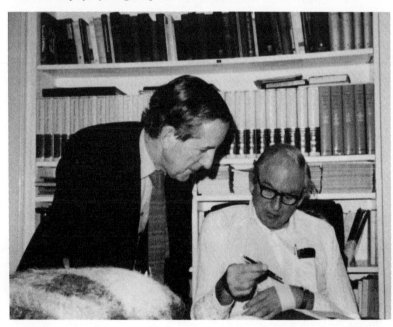

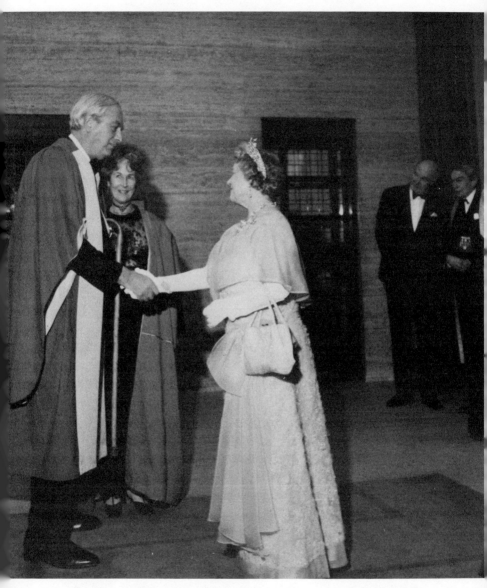

The Queen Mother, chancellor of London University, has just conferred an honorary doctorate on Peter. I am on his left, to steady him as he shakes hands without the support of his walking stick.

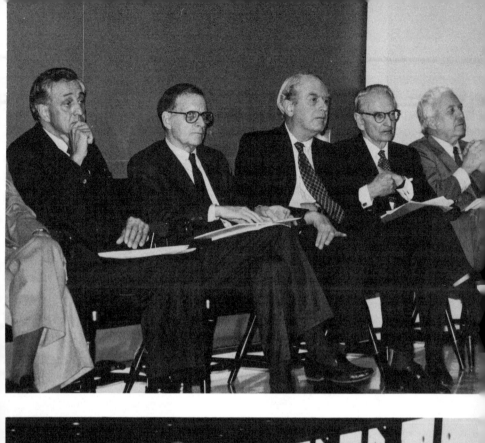

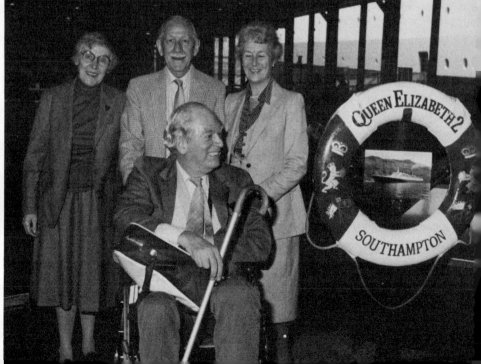

ON THE FACING PAGE: *Above, The platform at Sloan-Kettering Institute, New York, at the degree ceremony, March 19, 1980, the day before Peter had his second stroke: (left to right) Robert Good, Lewis Thomas, Peter, Laurance Rockefeller, and Ted Batey.*

Below, October 1984. Dorothy and Jerry Lawrence are seeing us off after Peter's last lectures in America. He had planned a restful voyage home, but the engines failed on the second day, and the ship rolled so badly that the captain begged the passengers not to distribute themselves all on one side of the vessel.

Golden wedding party, February 27, 1987.

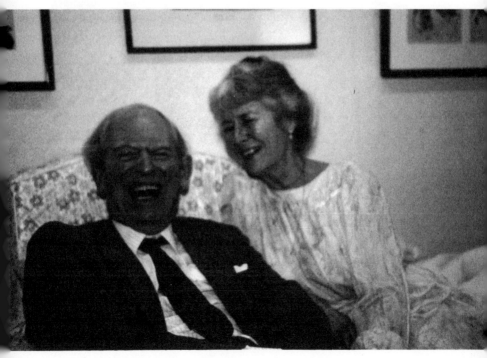

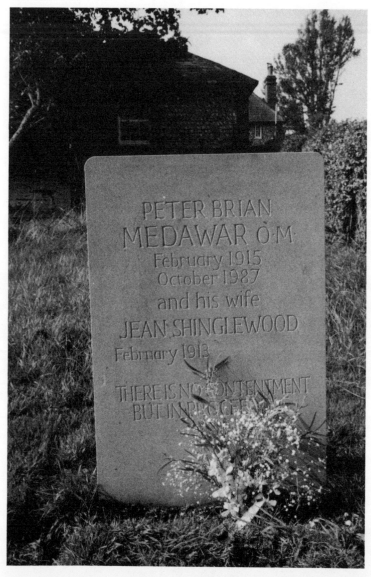

PETER BRIAN
MEDAWAR O·M·
February 1915
October 1987
and his wife
JEAN SHINGLEWOOD
February 1913

THERE IS NO CONTENTMENT
BUT IN PROCEEDING

*The headstone in Alfriston churchyard, Sussex, carved by Ralph
Beyer.*

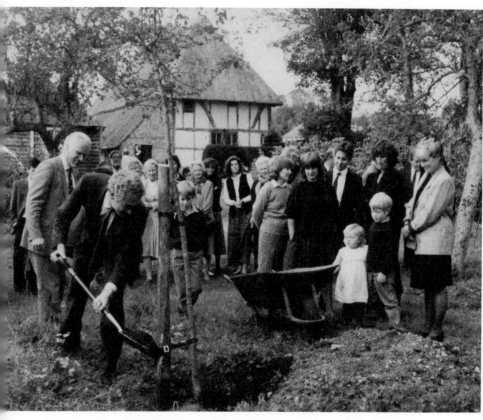

Our son Charles is helping to plant the first tree of the Medawar Memorial Grove at Alfriston, Sunday, October 1988, on the first anniversary of Peter's death. In the group are family and friends who have given donations to the National Trust for a tree in Peter's memory.

he would have chosen anyway. He now had a spotlessly clean laboratory—in University College the windows had had to be sealed up, to keep out dirt and other foreign bodies. As soon as he moved to Mill Hill, he spent thought and time in designing the placing of everything he needed for the grafting experiments, so that no time was wasted in rummaging for an instrument during an operation.

He took me to see his lab when it was finished. He was delighted with everything—his lab, his equipment, his colleagues, his book-lined office and his super secretaries Pauline Townend and Joy Heys. At Mill Hill there was no need to go to the animal house on Sunday to make sure that the mice had all they needed, because the animal houses were looked after by Jack Platts, the head of the Animal Husbandry Division. Jack set standards of care and efficiency which were envied, admired and imitated wherever animal husbandry was practised. He and Peter liked and amused each other, both as colleagues and as members of the Mill Hill cricket team.

Peter organised the responsibilities of running the National Institute in three and a half days—the other two and a half were sacred to research. Many human problems had to be solved and he thought that the administrative difficulties were pale by comparison. In almost any sample of one hundred people in the UK, one is likely to be a depressive or just plain difficult, and of the two hundred people at Mill Hill, there were at least two who came quite often to see Peter, in states of mild persecution or despair. Peter was good at listening attentively and he empathised to the extent of declaring that he too had bouts of depression; when he was in them, he said, he would do only routine work—washing glassware, cataloguing or some "banausic" job. At this word the visitor's eyebrows would be raised in query, and Peter explained the meaning—"fit for a labourer." Then they would both laugh and talk some more until whoever it was went away, encouraged perhaps by example.

The routine of the day hardly varied. One of the Institute's drivers picked him up in time to get him to Mill Hill before 9:00 a.m. and called for him again at the end of the day to arrive home for dinner at seven. When he got home he didn't want to unwind with a glass of wine and discuss the day's problems; he wanted to get on with the meal and then with the next item—work on the current lecture or a book review or taping some of his collection of gramophone records, stopping every now and then to repeat and conduct favourite passages from Wagner or Beethoven; or we might read or watch a TV programme. Once a month at least friends came to a meal or we dined with them or went to the theatre, cinema or opera.

Peter's views on hospitality agreed with Mr. John Knightley's in Jane Austen's novel *Emma,* who (on the way to dine out at his brother's house) grumbled: "A man must have a very good opinion of himself when he asks people to leave their own fireside . . . for the sake of coming to see him. The folly of not allowing people to be comfortable at home, and the folly of peoples' not staying comfortably at home when they can. . . ."

So, when we entertained at Mount Vernon House, he expected high standards. We sometimes sat twenty old and new friends at five round tables, four people at each, and by laying out five sets of everything beforehand, Peter and Charles were able to turn the L-shaped drawing room into a dining room in under five minutes. By now I was a decent cook, the wine came from the Wine Society, the company was good, and nobody seemed sorry that they had left the comfort of their own fireside.

One day Peter proposed that we should stop in Bermuda for a few days' holiday, on the way to a meeting of the American College of Physicians in Atlantic City where he was to be made an

honorary Fellow. I thought this was a wonderful idea. We rented
a cottage belonging to the Pink Beach Hotel, near enough to the
sea to hear the breakers on the shore. The place was idyllic, the air
was soft and smelt of jasmine and stephanotis. I hoped Peter would
unwind, but saw, almost with indignation, that the first time we
went down to the beautiful pink sand beach, he brought out a huge
volume from the Royal Society and began reading. However, we
swam when he'd read enough and we played tennis in the afternoon. His energy was enormous; after three sets (he as if his court
was double and mine single), he said, "Now what shall we do?" I
had been thinking of sinking into one of the recliners on the terrace
by the cottage, but instead we bicycled half round the island—and
it was actually refreshing. Arum lilies grew wild and breezes from
the sea were exactly the right temperature.

When he was made a honorary Fellow of the American College
of Physicians, Peter joked that this privilege allowed him to put up
a plate and to "practice medicine to the danger of the great American public." He stayed on till the end of the meetings. I went to
visit Charles, who was studying linguistics at the University of
Indiana at Bloomington. Charles had been the most untidy boy I
ever met. Now he had a small apartment and was as clean and
welcoming as any mother could wish. Loulie was by this time
earning her living in Chicago and she flew over for a quick visit.
They got on well and I was very proud of them both.

Peter got back to London before I did. On the day I arrived
home, I learnt that we were invited that evening to dine with Mr.
and Mrs. Cecil King in Cheyne Walk. Cecil King was at this time
a powerful newspaper baron. I think this was the first time I realised how sought after Peter had become. The other guests were
Lord and Lady Drogheda and Lord and Lady Devlin. The pooled
talents of the men would have equipped ten ordinary men; and the
women were remarkable too—Ruth King had initiated and organised the National Youth Orchestra and Lady Drogheda was an

accomplished pianist. I was too interested in the conversation and the surroundings to feel tired from the Atlantic flight, but I was surprised to learn that Cecil and Ruth King believed that a mysterious rash Mr. King sometimes suffered could be cured by a wise woman, operating from a distance, merely by handling some article of his clothing.

The Droghedas invited us to their box at Covent Garden the next week. This is the perfect way to enjoy opera. You reach the box by private, red-carpeted stairs and are welcomed by a beautifully mannered "flunkey." He shows you into an ante room where you meet your host and other guests—almost always people you would like to meet, a baritone, a writer, or the Cabinet secretary. On one side of the room is a dinner table set for eight and a smaller table for glasses and bottles of every variety. Opposite the dinner table are heavy red curtains, screening the interior of the box, the view of the auditorium and stage beyond it. In the box is a velvet chaise-longue. On it, with the aid of a mirror on the wall, King Edward VII used to sport with a pretty lady while keeping an eye on the progress of the opera.

In the first interval you emerge from the fantasy of the opera to the reality of dinner, waiting to be served. All the time-keeping is done by the head flunkey, so the host is alerted by a discreet whisper when it is time to wind up the conversation and return to the box for the next act.

The day after the night at the opera, Peter flew to New York. Three days later he was back playing bridge with his Mama and friends, and two days after that he came with me to Cambridge where the undergraduates were organising a meeting to raise funds for the Family Planning International Campaign. I don't remember what sort of talk I gave but I remember Peter's contribution. "Why," he asked, "since it is obvious that numbers of people grow at compound interest, and resources for them cannot grow at all, is there so much passionate antipathy to taking means to achieve a balance between human numbers and human needs?" His answer was, "Because the idea is *New.*" I had never thought of this, or its implications, and as far as I know, nobody else had either.

That summer of 1965 Peter played in seven village cricket matches. He loved the game, even when he made hardly any runs or was clean bowled. He loved the companionship and the expeditions, mostly to Sussex or Cambridge villages with a scratch team called the Trojans; he called them the Mendicant Musicians—of whom the conductor Colin Davis was the best known. Peter's height gave him a great advantage as a bowler. His run up ended in a flurry of small steps before he launched the ball, wearing an expression of grim concentration which I thought should paralyse the batsman. But this was real cricket, village cricket, without pressure from national honour or television commentators, and the players soon knew each other and everybody enjoyed themselves.

In cricket the tempo is not andante. Periods of intense concentration and activity alternate with wary idleness for the players, and the spectators can do as they like—live every moment of the game, shouting "Howzatt" a second before anyone else, or drowse in deck chairs under the brims of their Panama hats. In the background is the countryside, usually lush because of the rain, the smell of bruised grass and cows in the next field, cawing of rooks and clatter of crockery where lunch and pints of beer are being got ready by the wives and friends of the host side.

This year Margaret Pyke asked me to speak at the annual conference of the Family Planning Association to the eight hundred delegates in Church House in London. I knew what I had to say, but I was acutely nervous about standing up and saying it. Peter coached me. He recommended saying the following, every night before going to sleep: "When the time comes, I shall be calm, cool and collected." When the time did come, I stood up and as I opened my mouth I became detached from the person who was speaking.

How is she managing? I thought, and listened to her speaking, quite calmly. After that initiation I didn't mind other occasions so much, though I always took great trouble with what needed saying.

By 1965 two of our four children were independent. Caroline was studying for an M.A. in experimental psychology at Philadelphia under the benevolent eye of Hilary Koprowski, director of the Wistar Institute. That summer in America she married a fellow student from Cambridge, Peter Loizos, now a social anthropologist, rather too coolly we thought; we hoped for the best, but the marriage did not flourish and ended a few years later.

After a year studying physics at Peter's old college, Magdalen, in Oxford, Charles went to read linguistics at Bloomington University. He was one of ten selected to go to Moscow to polish up his Russian. Charles was an object of suspicion in the Moscow of those days, and no wonder. He was the son of a well-known scientist and had been at Oxford. So why had he gone to an American university, specialised in Russian and then come on to Russia? He was followed everywhere, rather inefficiently, and gave the "tail" a hard time by agilely dodging him.

We were lucky that although the children were abroad, they were extremely good letter-writers. Their style resembled Peter's—it was as if they were talking to us, and what they wrote was always interesting.

In June, the post brought a letter from the Prime Minister asking if Peter would accept the order of knighthood which he was proposing to recommend to the Queen. Some people prefer, for all sorts of reasons, not to be knighted, but we were not among them. The only person not at first delighted was Mrs. Brown, our daily and invaluable housekeeper since 1953. "I'll never be able to say, 'Sir Peter or Lady Medawar,' " she said, "never." But she did, or rather as soon as she saw there was no change in us. I noticed that the telephone operators at the National Institute were very delighted and quick off the mark. It was "Yes, Sir Peter," and "No, Sir Peter," on the day of the announcement.

Titles in England provoke a sort of love/hate reaction, half approving and half commonsense. Once I was being served in a country restaurant by an Italian maitre d' who actually hoped that the other diners would hear that he was serving a lady. "May I pour your wine, m'lady?" he said, and then, a moment later, reverting to his vernacular, "a spot of vino?" Four years later, when Peter was in hospital, the whole ward could hear when a nurse was attending to and requiring the co-operation of "Sir Peter."

On 16 November the Queen held an investiture at Buckingham Palace. Peter really became Sir Peter, and we celebrated by going to lunch at the Ritz. The surroundings and occasion were perfect, but Peter complained that the food wasn't up to the occasion and it really wasn't.

Soon after, while we were having dinner with Sir Philip and Lady Hendy, Sir Philip as Director of the National Gallery asked Peter if he would like to be invited to become a member of the Board of Directors. At this time Peter was longing to be invited to join the Board at Covent Garden Opera, where his knowledge of opera might have been useful, so he declined, wisely I thought, because his talents were not visual and he had too much to do already; but it was good to be asked.

Early in 1966 when I went to answer the telephone, a man's voice asked to speak to Dr. Medawar. There had been quite a few reporters wanting Peter's views on the after life, bimetalism, or cures for cancer, so I replied cautiously, "It depends who you are." The voice said, modestly, "Well, this is James Perkins and I am the President of Cornell." I could only laugh and say, "All right," and he then kindly added that he wished his wife would protect him in the same way. His call was to invite Peter to visit Cornell

University as a "professor at large." Peter accepted with pleasure and we arranged to go to Cornell in November.

We stayed there in the Statler Inn at which students were trained in hotel management. What a change from the tired, bored staff at the Seymour Hotel in New York where we had sometimes stayed. There, when I rang down to the desk to ask for help with the bags, an exasperated operator just said, "Yeah?" At the Statler Inn an eager voice asked, "Can I help you, ma'am?"

While Peter visited laboratories and talked to students, entertainment was laid on for visiting ladies. I regret that the only event I can remember is a rather comic lesson in flower arrangement demonstrated by a large lady and her small husband. His job was to hand her coloured squares of material, from a suitcase, to act as background for her compositions (I thought all of them were pretty awful). After a few designs the lady said she was going to demonstrate a "monochromatic" arrangement. She stopped and looked enquiringly at the audience. "Now, does anyone know what monochromatic means?" Several ladies, but not all, eager to please teacher, held up and waved their hands like schoolgirls. "I know, I know, choose me." I kept quiet, wanting to remember the accents to amuse Peter afterwards. Twenty years later James Perkins came to stay with us and the story still made us laugh.

By 1966, whenever Peter was invited to lecture in America, Canada, or Europe, he replied that he was of course delighted to be asked but that he did not now travel without the company of his wife—adding that he would perfectly understand if the University's funds would not run to the double expense. As far as I know they never refused and I was able to divert some of the strains of travel from Peter. He thought I was a good aide-de-camp—until I left one of his suitcases behind. Luckily, on this occasion, in Minneapolis, our host was Dr. John Najarian, as tall as Peter and built like the footballer he actually was. Peter borrowed clothes

from him and for the first time in his life had pyjamas that were
too big for him.

One year he was invited to accept an honorary degree from
Montreal, and he accepted on the usual terms. As we flew over
Canada and came in to land, we saw that we were entering a white
world, covered in thick snow; moments later, when the first trees
appeared on the outskirts of the city, Peter said, "My God. Everything is *en gelée!*" and so it appeared. Every twig and branch was
encased in clear ice and occasionally, as the wind moved the
branches, the mould cracked and splintered and the sun shone
minute rainbows through the splinters as they fell.

Peter was duly awarded an honorary degree and was asked to
give an uplifting address to the newly fledged graduates; in spite
of his frequent jeering at what he called "onward and upward"
addresses, he produced the right note of encouragement, humour
and relevance. At the finale of the ceremony the honorary graduates stood for applause on the platform, holding their parchment
degrees in elegant cardboard tubes. At the height of the applause
Peter looked down at me from the platform, raised his eyebrows,
lifted the tube to his ear and shook it for contents, as a child tests a
cracker.

There was a dinner that evening and endless drinks before it.
Normally, I stuck beside Peter to help him resist drinking too many
Martinis or Gibsons, pressed on him by kind hostesses. This time
I was led away to be introduced to a large circle of guests. By the
time I got back, Peter had drunk three Gibsons. I thought his eyes
were wandering a bit, and no wonder. "I am absolutely sloshed,"
he murmured as we sat down. He had to reply for the guests in an
after-dinner speech and I wondered if, when the time came, it
would be prudent of me to faint. On second thoughts I found a
waiter who constantly filled Peter's glass with water, and with this
and the adrenalin provided by the occasion he performed so well
that nobody realised what had been going on.

One February Peter returned to New York to be made a member of the New York Academy of Sciences, an honour he much enjoyed. The next month he flew to Reed College in Oregon to take part in a symposium on the Sanctity of Life. At this conference, Mr. Norman St. John Stevas, a Roman Catholic and later Minister for Education, spoke about the dangers of birth control, illustrating them by what is known as the Beethoven story. One doctor tells another of a recent case "about the termination of pregnancy. I want your opinion. The father was syphilitic, the mother tuberculous. Of the four children born, the first was blind, the second died, the third was deaf and dumb, the fourth was also tuberculous. What would you have done?" "I would have ended the pregnancy." "Then you would have murdered Beethoven," triumphantly replies the first doctor.

Peter's contribution to the Sanctity of Life theme followed directly after this dramatic story. In it he pointed out that, as each child conceived on any one occasion belongs to a vast cohort of possible children, every abstention from intercourse may also prevent the conception of a Beethoven. This idea sobered a lot of the audience.

Later on when we were in Liège, where Peter had been invited to adjudicate on the Prix Franchi, we stayed in the Fondation Universitaire, a rather austere and old-fashioned building. We planned to have dinner by ourselves that evening, having learnt to appreciate the quality of Belgian cooking. As we were getting ready, there was a knock on the door and a silver salver was presented, on which was lying a fat envelope. When we picked it up, it crackled—it contained enough new Belgian francs to eat even a Belgian-sized meal. And when we said we were planning to dine out, a car arrived to drive us to a nearby restaurant—the car was so long and the restaurant so nearby that Peter said we could have got there by getting in at the back of the car and out at the front. The restaurant was quiet and becomingly lit; we sat on green velvet seats surrounded by banks of pink and scarlet azaleas. Everything was delicious and because the number of the bank notes was greater than expected for an honorarium, I felt I could order Crèpes Suzette. All the ritual of rubbing lumps of sugar on the zest of oranges was expertly performed in front of us while we sipped Pouligny Montrachet ("You must pronounce the t in the middle," Peter said knowledgeably, and I was by then in no mood to doubt him). Finally we asked for the bill, having calculated that we had eaten most of the notes. *"Ah Monsieur,"* said the Maître d'Hôtel, *"c'est tout arrangé,"* and so it was, even to the imaginary walk back through the waiting car.

This luxurious Belgian week was followed by two weeks of comparative squalor. I flew to Chicago to help Loulie, who had just given birth to our first grandchild, Benjamin. She had invited me eight months earlier, and had delivered on the expected day. She and her doctor husband Len were living economically in two rooms while he was preparing for his final examinations. Len met me at the airport and we drove home in his VW beetle. We found Loulie in a miserable state, shivering and tearful. She had got out of bed to put the rubbish outside the apartment and the door had blown shut behind her. Benjamin had woken at the bang and started crying and she had no way of getting back inside. By the time she persuaded a surly janitor to come up from his basement with his keys, she was imagining that Benjamin was in danger of choking to death and was shivering with cold as well as fright.

Len and Loulie slept in a double bed in a bedroom the size of a cupboard, off the living room. I slept on a sofa and kept my suitcase under it. Benjamin slept soundly in a cot, near me. He was a long, thin baby and needed his feed from Loulie about every two hours. Besides the two rooms, the apartment had a shower, boxed off from the living room, and a kitchen into which black beetles from the flat below came up to eat cooking crumbs remaining on the gas stove. I cleaned it up, but they were difficult to deter. The landlady was Dickensian, disapproved of babies, and after a few days told Loulie that she would like them to leave. I went for a walk down the road, to cool my indignation, saw an apartment for rent and took it. It turned out to be a great improvement and they moved into it soon after I left.

During this fortnight Peter had engagements in Philadelphia and Boston so we kept in touch by telephone and rejoiced over Benjamin's safe arrival. By early May we were home in time for cricket matches, always the high point of Peter's summer.

19 June 1966 was the saddest day for me. On 9 June I had seen Margie (Margaret Pyke) onto the train for Scotland where she was to holiday with her cousin at Ardchattan Priory. Very early on the morning of the 20th, David rang us to say she had died there, of a brain haemorrhage. I still miss her, but I never forget her or her influence on me.

In the autumn of 1966 Peter went once again to Russia with Jim Gowans and Roy Calne on behalf of the British Council. Soviet hospitality was warm but the dead hand of politics was then cold on the work in the laboratories, and all three men were shocked when results were presented to them which were obviously tailored to fit political requirements. In his report to the British Council, Peter wrote of the clinical and experimental work on homotransplantation that "it would be hard to differentiate it objectively from fraudulence, for only successes are reported."

At the Institute of Animal Morphology, however, he was inspirited to find the same six scientists he and I had met and liked ten years earlier in Moscow—they were, he wrote, "open, jolly and younger looking."

NINE

The Crash, 1969

T HE YEAR 1969 started badly. Peter went to Boston and New York early in January. When he got home five days later he was unusually quiet, and I thought he was tired from the flight. That evening as he was undressing for bed and I was lying in the bath with the door open into the bedroom, I heard him say, "I think I've got cancer." I remember thinking, I must be sensible. I said as casually as I could, "Oh Peter, what makes you think that?" Still in the other room, he said in a strained voice, "Because I have a growth on my testicle." I got out of the bath and went to hug him and to make plans. We made an appointment with a surgeon next day and the diagnosis brought immediate relief—the "growth" was a cyst from which the fluid could be aspirated. Mr. Davis, the surgeon, recommended that the cyst should be removed, but Peter said he had no time for an operation. So the fluid was aspirated and the treatment relieved him of both pressure and anxiety. In my diary, that day, is a note in red ink, "Sick with relief." Actually I cooked a celebratory dinner of pheasant with butter, cream, Bramley apples and Calvados brandy.

The following weekend, Peter played squash, first with Charles and then with Alexander, and tired them both out—at least that was his claim, and I think they liked to allow it.

Peter's mother died in the spring. She had broken her hip the year before and had a failing liver. We installed her in a nursing home in Hampstead and bought a wheelchair for her convalescence. Peter came every day and made her laugh and we planned the date of her coming home. I was with her in the nursing home as she died quite unexpectedly from a cerebral haemorrhage. She died content: she had lived to watch Peter, on television, receive the Nobel Prize in Stockholm, to welcome her great-grandchildren, and she had told me that her days in our upstairs flat were the happiest in her life. She and Peter were friends as well as relatives, and they constantly amused each other with bridge, greatly exaggerated comic stories and family anecdotes, all of which he loved, and missed. But he had been a model son and although he was sad, he took more time in remembering her jokes than in mourning her death. He tried never to mope or brood about the inevitable and usually succeeded. He was anyway obliged to concentrate on his preparations for the meetings of the British Association over which he was to preside. Every night after supper he set up his typewriter in front of the fire and rattled down his ideas for one major presidential address and eleven small speeches.

I noticed about this period that from time to time Peter slipped his right hand into the left side of his jacket and held it away from his chest. When I asked him what the matter was, he said it was nothing—he felt he needed some hard exercise. After a few of these episodes I persuaded him to visit the President of the Royal

College of Physicians, Lord Rosenheim—an excellent physician and a very agreeable friend. Max examined Peter, found he had rather high blood pressure, and told him to take life more easily. At this time Professor (later Sir) James Black had not yet discovered that a drug which came to be called a beta-blocker could slow down the heart rate and regulate high blood pressure. The alternative was a drug that had unpleasant side effects. In 1969, medical opinion was divided on the subject of high blood pressure. Some held it always to be a pathological sign and others that it was part of an individual's make-up—some people were quite normal even if their pressure was high, so bringing it down might cause too much interference.

At this point Peter was not in a position to take life more easily, either by circumstances or temperament. I was very busy as chairman of the Family Planning Association, and with plans for setting up a suitable memorial to Margaret Pyke. Ever since her death in 1966, David and I had set our hearts on establishing something worthy of her life and work. We started a fund through the pages of the journal *Family Planning* and money began to come in from most of the eight hundred clinics all over the country, from the International Planned Parenthood Federation and from friends and relations. We decided to set up a model training centre for study and education in family planning. I wrote to Prince Philip to invite him to open it. His letter of acceptance came that summer. This acceptance was a landmark in the history of the family planning movement and Peter, busy though he was, shared my joy at the news. He had a great capacity for vicarious enjoyment and knew as well as I did how much good this royal patronage would do.

By the autumn all the preparations for the British Association meetings in Exeter were finished, and on 1 September Peter travelled to Exeter by train, leaving me to drive down in our new car two days later.

We stayed in the Judges' Lodgings, at Larkbeare in Exeter.

Judges on circuit expect their comforts, and in the absence of the judge we enjoyed them and the way his staff looked after us. A magnolia grandiflora grew right up to the first-floor bedroom window where we slept. In the dusk the flowers looked luminous; by the end of the week of our stay, the topmost buds had opened, and I leant out of the bedroom window to smell them. They were so close I could watch the tiny black insects creeping about in the velvety cup of petals, sipping the nectar. I did not know that this was the last evening I would ever have without anxiety for Peter's health or safety. By the end of the next fifteen hours, our life had been cruelly changed and could never be the same again.

After 7 September 1969 it never was the same again. Halfway through reading the lesson Peter collapsed in the Cathedral, an ambulance was called, and we were rushed to the Exeter Royal Infirmary. There the physician in charge, Dr. John Simpson, met us, and as he looked at Peter said, "I promise we won't undertake any heroic measures," a promise which confirmed my terrible fears. Once Peter had been admitted and I had been given a bed in the attic of the hospital, I remembered that three of our children were in France and might first learn of their father's stroke from a newspaper. I was grateful to a friend who kept the journalists at bay and delayed publication of the news until I could contact them. Our friend David Pyke had always said, "If anything is ever wrong with anyone in the family, get hold of Max Rosenheim." Lord Rosenheim was a lovely man, a superb physician, and Peter had already been to him for advice. A messenger reached him and he arranged to come to Exeter. When he arrived next day, he examined Peter carefully and decided that he should be transferred to the care of Dr. Michael Kremer in the Neurology Department of the Middlesex Hospital, in London. He realised that an operation was necessary to relieve the pressure from blood leaking into the tightly enclosed brain. As it had to be done, he wanted it done by Mr. John Andrew, in charge of Neurosurgery at the Middlesex. I packed up everything at the Judges' Lodgings in a dazed sort of hurry. Someone bought tickets and reserved a whole railway carriage—I ought to have asked who paid for it, but I forgot. Peter, still unconscious, arrived at the station in an ambulance on a stretcher; the men arranged it from corner to corner of the carriage.

The stretcher took up most of the room, and a nurse, a doctor and I fitted into what remained. I don't remember much about the journey except that I kept on either falling asleep or talking to Peter, in case he could hear and be reassured, and that the nurse and doctor were very kind. Caroline, David Pyke and the Middlesex ambulance met us at Paddington Station. We drove to the hospital and Peter was at once wheeled away to be prepared for the operation. Dr. Michael Kremer, the great and compassionate head of Neurology at the hospital, arrived and took charge.

He tucked my arm under his, walked me quickly into his office and began, matter of factly, to show me, on a model of the brain, where he thought the damage was, and what the prospects were. Peter's stroke had been in the right side of the brain, in the frontal lobe. Michael Kremer pointed to the small area that controlled the movements of the leg, then, further on, the arm, hand and fingers, and the eye. A blood vessel had ruptured, under the high blood pressure, depriving the cells of oxygen, without which they died. Pressure was building up inside the skull—a big clot had formed and was pressing on other parts of the brain and affecting his breathing. The clot had to be removed.

Given a choice and if you are right-handed, it would be preferable to have a stroke in the right half of the brain because it controls the left side of the body, and not the right where the speech centre lies. If one could choose between two evils, perhaps one would opt for the type of damage done by a clot in the blood vessels, and not by a rupture in which blood seeps into the brain and damages other areas as the pressure increases. Perhaps the least preferable sort of stroke occurs in a deep-lying area of the brain where it can cause behavioural changes which deform the original character.

The day after the operation Michael Kremer behaved as doctors are popularly held not to behave; he drew me into the picture and asked me to help rouse Peter. I moistened my lips, combed my hair and tried: "Come on, Peter. Open your eyes and tell me where you are." His eyes opened slowly. He was very tired. He announced, in a weak voice, "Entire visual field agreeably occupied," and shut his eyes again. This freshly coined phrase could have been delivered only by Peter and only if his brain was undamaged in the essential areas. I felt delight and relief and needed to weep.

During the next two weeks he improved, very slowly. Recovery from a stroke depends on many factors: its size, where it is in the brain, the age and temperament of the patient, whether he or she prefers living to dying—and on the quality of the nursing care. In Campbell-Thompson Ward of the Middlesex there were three special graces: Sister Shirley Kean, Staff Nurse Carrie and Staff Nurse Margaret. They were all lovely to look at and they cared for each patient as well as nursing them. When there was a disaster in the bed, there were no pursed lips, but solicitude for the misery and embarrassment of the patient. Furthermore, they let me help and we became friends. I came every afternoon, emptied bottles, picked up things dropped from beds and generally tried to be useful. Sister Kean relied on my knowledge of Peter to help her understand what he wanted. At one point he was confused and kept asking how all his mice were. Instead of worrying about the occasional hallucinations, she asked me what was bothering him, and I explained that the mice were real and lived in his laboratory, and he was wishing he could be with them.

Peter had a stroke large enough to kill, in a part of his brain where it disabled the left half of each eye and his left arm and leg.

He was fifty-four, had a very decided preference for remaining alive, and was in a neurosurgical ward where the care could not have been better.

He lay flat in his bed, could not lift his head and had to be turned from one side to the other by two of the strongest nurses, every two hours. His voice was reduced to a grey whisper, but he was conscious. His sense of order persisted. Everything he needed, clock, push-bell for summoning a nurse, water glass and handkerchief, all had to be laid out on the locker beside him, and all in the same order.

When the time came for physiotherapy, his six foot four inches needed three supporters. As I came into the ward I saw Peter, trying to stand, like a fallen crumpled giant, supported by two Valkyrie-sized physiotherapists; another was on her knees on the floor, gently pulling at a bandage attached to his powerless left leg. Later that day I asked Peter how the first session had gone. He smiled. "I managed to scrape some of them off on the larger bits of furniture," he said. He had also noticed the nurse on her knees and suggested that I should buy her some new tights in case she had laddered the ones she was wearing.

The physiotherapy was done against a background of immense exhaustion. After some time I discovered that Peter was routinely given two whole tablets of Mogadon (Nitrazepam) every night— the dose being apportioned to his size. Nobody had asked if he were particularly sensitive to drugs. Later, at home, I found that one eighth of a tablet gave him a good long night. So, in the morning in hospital he felt, as he called it, "knackered," and when the time came for physiotherapy he could barely stand.

I came into the ward unexpectedly one day and heard the head of the Physio Department exclaim, from behind the curtains round Peter's bed, with a mixture of anger and disgust, "This is ridiculous!" as Peter fell back on the bed instead of remaining standing. At the time, I felt righteous anger, but although the remark should not have been made, I have since learnt how appallingly difficult it is for a healthy helper to restrain such feelings in all circumstances. It is not too hard to be patient and understanding when some disaster happens—like having got your loved one into a clean suit and he can't get to the lavatory in time; but other minor happenings, such as an obstinate refusal to recognize what is perfectly clear to oneself, have the power to irritate outrageously— and of course inexcusably. I have felt it myself and seen it happen in the hospital ward. Once Peter decided he wanted to "go upstairs," when he could not even stand. I tried explaining that it wasn't yet possible, but would be in time. This didn't work, and when he finally glared at me and said, "It's only *you* that are stopping me," I wanted to throw the pillow at him. I can't remember what I said but it certainly wasn't kind, and the memory made me weep. Of course we made it up, but some self-disgust remains. I gradually learnt that reason, in these situations, is no good; distraction and a sense of humour are.

Another time, in another hospital ward, I watched a devoted father daily gently ministering to his helpless son's needs, feeding him, wiping up the dribble and trying to communicate with him. One day, as the son again refused to swallow, the father's temper flared and he said things he probably couldn't bear to remember; but he was back next day, as caring as before.

After a bad stroke, unless the effects are transient, feeding is a problem and meals are not what they used to be. When Peter was helped out of bed and into the easy chair I had brought in from home, meals were set in front of him on the sort of bed table that swings over the lap from an adjustable stand. He could not lift his head, and the sight of his efforts, with saliva running down his chin onto the plate, was a misery. I didn't say anything, but he felt what I was feeling. He pulled his head up, gave a rather twisted smile, and said, "I always was a dirty feeder, you know."

The dribbling improves as the neck muscles strengthen, but

when one side of the mouth is paralysed, it is impossible to remember that it probably needs wiping. This is not a tragedy, but it is hard for the helper to tolerate, because it is an outward and visible sign of a disability whose effects one is trying to get around. Constant reminders to wipe have little effect and are bound to irritate both parties. Sometimes it helps to put the napkin on the left paralysed side; then the head turns to look where it is and the side of the mouth gets wiped as the head turns back.

About two months after Peter was admitted to the Middlesex he developed a persistent headache. One night there was a crisis, with high blood pressure and delirium. Mr. John Andrew was hastily summoned and decided to operate again. When he re-opened the site he found a slowly developing abscess. He cleared it and started Peter on a course of antibiotics.

Some people felt this should never have happened—someone should be blamed. Why had sterile precautions with the tubes draining the operation site not been more rigorous? I think I felt more charitable only because I had had some experience in the Oxford Pathology Laboratory of the difficulties of preventing infection. Living conditions in the ward cannot be kept as they are in an operating theatre.

At any rate Peter slowly recovered again, but there was no recovery for the left hand and forearm, the left leg was very weak, and there was no improvement in the sight of the left side of each eye. His long legs always had a tendency to bend backward, and now the curve on the left knee was worse because the thigh muscle was weak and reduced from lying in bed. The physios made a sling for the left arm with a pocket in a belt for his hand to rest in, and this relieved some of the weight from the left shoulder which had become painful. It hurt a great deal, but gradually improved with physiotherapy.

During Peter's time in hospital, friends and acquaintances sorted themselves into those who did him good and those who didn't.

The first lot rang home first to find out whether a visit would be welcome and if so what time, when, and for how long. When they came, they remembered that Sister was in charge, asked permission to visit, and when they saw Peter they encouraged him— "Goodness, how much better you look. You *are* making progress"—or some such remark. Encouragement never failed to have a good effect, especially if accompanied by grapes, truffles or really funny anecdotes. I used to bring him a leek and potato soup in a Thermos, hoping it would make up for my inability, at the time, to think of funny stories. Peter looked forward to it. "Where is my *nerve* soup?" he enquired, if I hadn't managed to bring it on time.

After five months in hospital, from September 1969 to March 1970, it was time to try what improvement might be achieved at a rehabilitation centre. Peter has given his version of the time he spent in the Atkinson Morley rehabilitation centre in South London in his *Memoir of a Thinking Radish*. What I remember most clearly is the dispiriting atmosphere of the place. After the care and understanding we had been given in the Middlesex Hospital, I guessed that we might find anywhere else inferior, so tried not to make critical comparisons; but this was not possible, because the contrasts were too large and too painful to be smiled away.

The first change I noticed was that Peter's useless left arm had been removed from the Middlesex design of sling, and where his shoulder had been normally rounded, the arm had dropped, leaving a skin-covered hollow between the end of the clavicle and the head of the humerus. Instead of encouragement from pretty nurses, I was made to feel unwelcome by the male nurses; Peter was nearly always weeping when I arrived, and wept when I left. He asked me to bring him a keepsake, for when I wasn't there. I bought the largest wedding ring I could find; but I had to have it made even larger. He wore it and rubbed it for comfort, and said it helped.

Though it is well known that the main factor in the making of an atmosphere is the quality of the organiser at the top, until now I had not fully appreciated how true this is. I decided to bring Peter home. I consulted Michael Kremer and he agreed, so I made an appointment with the director of the hospital and explained that I wanted to cut Peter's stay short. "On your own head be it," he replied indifferently. I managed not to tell him that the way he ran the hospital was on his head. We left the next day.

On the way home, on a clear road, I forgot the speed limit in my eagerness to get Peter back and drove a little over 30 miles an hour. Almost at once we were overtaken by a police car, driven by a heartless policeman who served me with a fine.

I can't remember the details of how we managed at home, but at that time the British United Provident Association paid for a nurse who looked after Peter at night. Now, BUPA resembles car insurers: if you have had an accident, and claim for it, you lose your bonus. In similar fashion one stroke deprives you of nursing help for another, even though you may always have paid your full annual premiums.

When we first got home, Peter had to use the kitchen sink for a bathroom because he couldn't get upstairs and I turned the adjacent dining room into a bedroom. Later, we tried to manage the stairs, both heaving, panting and pulling on the bannisters. As we reached the landing I remember thinking, Now it's my turn to go to bed. Peter was in no state to agree. But after that we began to think of the stairs as a form of physiotherapy when we used them twice a day. The exercise gradually strengthened the muscles of the left leg so that he could walk again. We were glad we had not taken advice to move to a flat where this exercise was not built in.

As spring and warmer weather came, we started to consider that we might manage a holiday. Friends considered it too—among them, Victor Rothschild. He asked me to breakfast and proposed the most imaginative and generous idea, that his holiday house in Barbados should be ours, he said. He was working in Cambridge, so we could accept his offer without inconveniencing him and his family. When Eugene Lance and other friends in America who had either worked with Peter or knew of his work and wanted to help heard of this plan for convalescing, they organised a Get Well gift in the form of two tickets to Barbados, on a Geest Line banana boat.

By May we had travelled by train to the boat and were comfortably installed in the owner's double cabin, on our way across the Atlantic to Barbados. At this time Peter could just manage to walk, but it was very difficult for him because his left knee bent backwards, and either kept him lower on the left side or performed like an ageing catapult. He could also see just enough to read, and tried to read Jane Austen to me once we were safely in our bunks at night; it was a very gallant effort, but his voice was very slow and without much volume or expression, and he soon tired and fell asleep.

The worst moment of the voyage was when a storm blew up. I wanted to be sick and so did Peter. He had to get to the washbasin and I had to support him to it, over a heaving floor, without being sick myself on the way. I remember noticing that a really desperate duty can override even the demands of a rebellious stomach. The storm didn't last, and when the sun came out we basked in it. After two days we attempted a dip in the swimming bath, helped by a lifebelt on a rope held by two sailors. It was not a success. The water sloshed too strongly up the sides of the pool and Peter's helpless left leg was at risk, so it was a relief when we got him out safely.

In Barbados, transport had been laid on to the Rothschild house and help arranged; before long we were sitting on the verandah built of white coral stone, inhaling fragrant warm air and sipping long rum drinks. We looked straight out over a fringe of palms to a private beach of white sand, up and down which the clearest cool water rippled loudly enough to be heard indoors.

Dinner was served by Braithwaite, Victor's butler, and we went early to bed soon after he had left. Peter hadn't seemed unusually tired, so I slept without anxiety. At about 6:00 a.m. the next morning I was woken by the sound of choking. Peter's eyes were rolled up and he was convulsing and shaking the bed. All I could remember from first aid was that "the patient must not be allowed to swallow the tongue." Peter's mother had died in such a seizure while I had been with her. I managed to get two of my fingers between Peter's teeth and held him as firmly as I could, murmuring whatever came into my head: "Take it easy, darling—it'll soon be better—it'll soon be over." It wasn't over for about three minutes, seemingly endless, but he was alive. He then slept very deeply. I couldn't, though I felt extremely tired.

At about eight o'clock Braithwaite came back to prepare breakfast and I tried to explain, without much success, what had happened. I decided to ring the local English doctor. Before I could contact him, Dr. Vernon Nickel and his wife arrived. Dr. Nickel, a distinguished American orthopaedic surgeon, was a friend of Eugene Lance and had been on holiday when he heard of Peter's stroke. He generously decided to visit us in Barbados on his way home. He ran a rehabilitation centre in California, called Rancho de los Amigos. There patients were treated by a team of orthopaedic surgeons, physicians, physiotherapists and orthotists. Vernon Nickel arrived just at the right time. I was shaken by the experience of the early morning seizure and about the foreseeable future. "But seizures are quite normal," he told me, "and the patient need feel no worse after than before."

He examined Peter carefully. When he had finished he said, "This is what we would term a moderate stroke. What you need is a good assessment of what can't be helped and what can. You need a good splint for the left leg to prevent the backward bend of the knee—this will help the walking. There is a very good man, Mr. Tuck at the Royal National Orthopaedic in London, you should go to see him." This line of talk was exactly what we both needed. The Nickels pooh-poohed my gratitude, said they had often meant to visit Barbados and were glad of the chance to meet Peter. I never forget how much their visit helped us both.

I did not mention the seizure to Peter. He had enough to put up with without thinking, I've had an epileptic fit as well as a stroke. He was tired and quiet for the next few days. He tried to write and was obsessional about getting on with what he wanted to get down— but the writing was illegible, even to him, and this frustrated him horribly and was sickening to see.

Loulie was then living in America with two small children and I was able to telephone her. She decided to join us and I was very glad she did; but it was sad being in a sort of Paradise, yet not in a position to be happy. Everything was beautiful—Loulie, the children, the climate, the house, the private beach, the rum punches, someone to make them, cook, and wash up afterwards—but all shadowed by constant anxiety. And Peter was unable to enjoy any of it.

Victor Rothschild's kindness extended to his insisting that he wanted me to make a report on the family planning services of the island. So, while Loulie stayed with Peter, I went round the clinics for an hour or so a day, collected attendance and drop-out figures and wrote a short account of what I learnt. I hope Victor had time to read it. Anyway it was short, and it distracted and interested me.

After a week I rang Michael Kremer to ask his advice about how to come home, and on balance, he thought it was better to come by air rather than take the longer sea trip. I asked the English doctor what to do if Peter had another seizure on the plane. He gave me a phial and hypodermic. There was fortunately no need for it, because it turned out to contain a dose which patients were given if a seizure did not stop after a few minutes.

When we got home, I consulted Michael Kremer about Peter's

blood pressure and the possibility of more seizures. I still hadn't mentioned them to Peter. When I told Michael about how I had tried to stop Peter swallowing his tongue during the attack, he smiled and said, "Jean, you only have eight fingers. All you need do is to keep Peter's head up and this will save both his tongue and your fingers."

After the blood pressure had been at the normal level of 130/90 for some months, I asked Michael Kremer if we could try reducing the dose of anti-hypertensive propanolol, otherwise how could anyone tell if it were necessary? He agreed, providing that I went on checking the pressure. I took six months to reduce the 70 mg he was taking down to none, and the pressure remained at 130/90.

The seizures were being treated with two drugs, mysolin and epanutin. They impaired Peter's ability to think and made his stomach lining ache. We began to wonder how to balance their disadvantages against the risk of another seizure. The seizures gradually became less violent and after one, in which Peter did not become unconscious, he asked me if he had fainted. I told him he had been having "blackouts," that they were now very slight and that Michael Kremer had said they would probably fade away. He then told me that he had, on some of these occasions, experienced what he called a "sense of impending dissolution," but that he had heard my voice through it and had felt safe. So perhaps the talking while he was convulsing had done us both good.

We took the risk of reducing the mysolin and epanutin—very gradually—and after the thirteenth seizure in April 1974 he had no more. Peter felt much better without drugs and I felt less anxious.

We were lucky in our medical friends. They understood Peter's need to go on working and what it was like for me to adapt to what an American friend called "the noo ball game." Our friend and general practitioner Dr. John Horder visited one day after Peter had had a setback. I was miserable. He asked, "Can I do anything for you, Jean?" I said, "Hold my hand," and this helped. I don't know how comfort could be taught in medical school, but sometimes a human handhold is better than a tranquilliser—and there is no half-life effect either.

By July 1970, ten months after the stroke, Peter decided to try to begin to work again as Director of the National Institute in Mill Hill. The driver came for him at 9:30 a.m. and brought him back at about 4:30. He arrived home with just enough strength to be helped to the sofa in the sitting room, and there he slept deeply for two to three hours. During this period his secretaries Pauline Townend and Joy Heys made it possible for him to keep up with the piles of correspondence from which all directors suffer. Because half of Peter's sight was gone, I checked almost all his home correspondence and was relieved to find how much he could do. What he could not do was read the first two or three words on the left side of the printed page, and when they contained "no" or "not" he naturally misread the sentence; otherwise he was coping extraordinarily well.

But the Medical Research Council became concerned that the responsibility of running their largest medical research institute might prove too much of a strain for Peter. It was decided to transplant him and those of his immediate colleagues who would accompany him to the newly built Clinical Research Centre (CRC) and regional hospital complex, out at Harrow on the Hill, ten miles from the centre of London. The following notice was pinned on the main notice board at Mill Hill:

DIRECTORSHIP OF NATIONAL INSTITUTE FOR
MEDICAL RESEARCH
STATEMENT FROM MEDICAL RESEARCH COUNCIL

Sir Peter Medawar wishes to be relieved of his responsibilities as Director of the National Institute for Medical Research in order to make his time available for research and writing.

Council have therefore agreed to transfer him from March 1st to a research post at the Clinical Research Centre.

Council wish to take this opportunity of expressing their deep gratitude to Sir Peter for making the National Institute for Medical Research a world centre in the field of immunology and for his contribution as a leader, loved and admired by those who worked for him. This leadership has enabled the highest standards to be maintained throughout the Institute. They also wish to put on record their great admiration for the way he has continued to bear his responsibilities in spite of the considerable physical handicaps left by his illness and they now wish him every success and happiness on his return to full-time research.

26th January 1971

This was a bad blow for Peter: he had for nine years delighted in his job at Mill Hill, but, as he said, he did see a lot of sense in the change. The blow was greatly softened by the presence of the friends and colleagues who chose to move with him.

Eugene Lance, a young and very successful orthopaedic surgeon in New York, had come over from America in 1962 with his family to work with Peter. Peter found him the brightest and most amusing colleague he had ever had, so when Eugene stayed on in spite on Peter's illness and was appointed head of the Division of Surgical Sciences out at the Clinical Research Centre, this was a tremendous encouragement. Then Dr. Elizabeth Simpson decided to come too. Peter wrote, "It was a source of particular pleasure to me that Dr. Elizabeth Simpson—one of the foremost immunologists in England—opted to join me. She added greatly to the scientific strength and what I called the mateyness of the little group of workers that now set up house in the CRC."* Lastly, but very importantly, Ruth Hunt and Joy Heys moved with Peter to Northwick Park. Ruth had worked with Peter as his research assistant and Joy had been Peter's second secretary at Mill Hill. Ruth's skill

*Memoir of a Thinking Radish, p. 163.

and patience were crucial to Peter, and so was Joy's ability to organise his papers, type his lectures, and generally see that the department and his working life ran smoothly.

During this time either Caroline, Charles, or Loulie came every Sunday for lunch or supper. We were lucky that, although all four children had gone to America to university, or to a job in Chicago, all three returned to settle in Hampstead within walking distance of us. Alexander, the youngest, was then still free-floating, feeling rather out of sympathy with us and our generation.

Peter later wrote of this period that "I felt as if my life had been transposed to a lower key . . . the great enemy of which I became acutely aware was tiredness, and I spent the working day longing for the evening to come and the working week longing for the weekend."* At David Pyke's suggestion we paid a visit to Sir Richard ("Dick") Bayliss—not for nothing had he been appointed as the Queen's physician. When he heard that Peter was taking the drug propanolol to control the blood pressure, he snorted indignantly and prescribed a newer version called metaprolol which did not cross over the blood barrier into the brain; this change brought a great relief. No wonder, as I discovered when at a conference in Austria I once carelessly swallowed one of Peter's propanolol pills in mistake for an aspirin to relieve a cold. In the morning I felt unable to move. My limbs and the rest of my body felt far away from my control and all I wanted to do was sleep. It was Peter who guessed what had happened, and the alarming diagnoses by medical friends at the conference of what was wrong with me were rapidly forgotten; but after that one pill it took me twenty-four hours to feel at all normal again.

By 1971 we could assess our hopes of progress: Peter was working again, without undue pressure, his walking was improving, his blood pressure was fine and he was off drugs—and beginning to write in his old style.

Memoir of a Thinking Radish, p. 160.

TEN

Progress, 1971

B Y JANUARY 1971 Peter felt strong enough to sit through Wagner's *Meistersingers*, at Covent Garden Opera House, and to take friends out for supper at Simpsons Restaurant, though not, mercifully, one after the other in the same evening. Next month we sat through *Götterdämmerung*—the first act alone lasts two and a half hours. Soon his stamina was up to a formal dinner. For his first public appearance, David Pyke invited us to dine at the Royal College of Physicians. The President paid a special tribute to Peter in his speech of welcome to the guests, and the applause from the physicians who knew what he had overcome gave him pleasure at the time and increased his confidence about the future.

A few months later he accepted an invitation to reply for the guests at a dinner in the Apothecaries Hall. His speech was clear and witty in a way that removed any anxiety the audience might have had about his preference for remaining alive or his ability to entertain. Recently, he explained, he had undergone "an examination of the state of the interior of his head." A young lady had placed "a sort of electric bonnet" over it and had urged him to tell her at once if he felt at all odd. "I shall know if you've fainted," she had assured him, "because *I* can see if your stomach drops." The shout of laughter showed him that he could still amuse an audience.

In the summer of 1971 Jill Spalding, a friend of mine and the Literary Editor of *Vogue,* asked if she could write an article about Peter, illustrated with a photograph taken by Lord Snowdon. Peter couldn't see much connexion between his writing and *Vogue* magazine, but he agreed, to please Jill, and he wrote a good article about scientific drive entitled "The Restless Endeavour." Lord Snowdon took the photograph from the garden outside, looking in at Peter, who was writing at the special large table I had fitted into the bay window of the sitting room. A geranium and our tabby cat Moppet also featured in the photograph. Peter looked tired, and when he saw the picture he said rather coldly that he supposed it was good of the cat.

Early in 1969, the year of Peter's stroke, when Dr. John Graham of the University of North Carolina had invited him to give the 1971 Merrimon Lectures, he had accepted. By the summer of 1971 we thought he could manage to give them. John Graham visited London in August and we invited him to have dinner with us at Simpsons. I remember asking him if he was a "proper doctor" or a scientific one. He was a real M.D., so I felt Peter would be safely looked after in Chapel Hill.

We decided to go to America on the *QE2* and to fly on to Chapel Hill from New York. Our idea was to take it easy on the boat and to practice walking round and round the deck. But almost as soon as we had settled down on board, I realised that Peter was planning to read the audience the lecture he had prepared—a thing he had never done before. His voice was still very underpowered, and if he had read his material out loud the audience might have fallen asleep. So instead of taking it easy and exercising round the deck we spent a lot of time turning the lecture into notes which Peter learnt. Another problem we realised as he practised was how to manage the choking emotion he felt for the quotations of beautiful seventeenth-century prose—since the stroke, the words caused real sobs no matter how often we rehearsed the passages. How could he (especially in his state) not be moved by Sir Thomas Browne, who described his generation as "ordained in the setting part of time"? "The great mutations of the world are acted," Browne wrote, and, "It is too late to be ambitious."

"You'll just have to prick yourself with this tie pin," I said matter of factly, and showed him a suitable pearl-headed pin in my handbag, made of gold and sharp enough not to hurt too much.

By the time the boat docked in New York, Peter felt more confident about giving the lecture and his voice had gathered strength from the exercises we practised every day of the voyage—roaring like lions, and hissing like snakes.

Dr. Jerry Lawrence, one of the original "visiting firemen," had promised to meet us at the dock in New York. Peter was nervous about how we would get off the *QE2,* but he need not have worried. Jerry had been a naval officer and I was sure that he would have all methods of disembarkation under tight control. Sure enough, the engines had barely stopped when there was a tap on the door, and as I opened it Jerry stood there saluting and smiling. Beside him were two strong interns from the New York University Hospital and on the quay a large car was waiting. From then on, Jerry and his wife Dorothy took over all arrangements. We had only to comply, and this relaxed behaviour and their thoughtfulness got us comfortably into the plane going to Chapel Hill in North Carolina.

When the plane landed in Chapel Hill, John Graham was standing at the bottom of the gangway with another two strong interns. We came down naval fashion, backwards, as Peter's sister Pamela had suggested, with Peter above me, while I gripped the handle of a stout orthopaedic belt round his waist. "Well," John Graham said between welcoming and laughing, "I often saw a man tied to his mother's apron strings but never before did I see a man attached to his wife by a big ole belt." We felt at home with this friendly jeering and the friendship has grown in the seventeen years since then. We stayed at the Grahams' house in the middle of the woods, Peter rested, and we felt safe in their care.

When the time came for the lecture, the theatre was packed; somebody told me every neurologist in town was attending, some of them out of curiosity to see how Peter would manage after the crippling stroke he had suffered.

I thought he managed brilliantly, and so did the audience. The lecture was on Science and Civilisation—and all the ideas and ilustrations in the roughly 6,000 words were clear, fresh and interesting. When he came to the "too late to be ambitious" passage, his voice almost disappeared into the back of his throat. I was sitting in the row immediately below the lectern. He glanced down at me and I mouthed *"Pin"* at him. His mood changed as fast as a child's and he recovered, smiled and continued more strongly, without using the pin. This first post-stroke visit to America might have been tiring. Instead, partly because we were surrounded by people who wanted to help, it had the opposite effect, as if he had swallowed strengthening medicine.

By 1972 we were managing a relatively normal life. Peter was driven daily to and from the Clinical Research Centre. He was still thinking of ingenious experiments, but with one hand and half of each eye out of commission his ability to carry out delicate procedures was very limited. At first Ruth Hunt tried to act as his left hand, working at a narrow operating table and sitting opposite

Peter. Soon, firmly but kindly, she explained that the results would be better if Peter did most of the thinking and she did all the handiwork. I admired this achievement of hers, because I remembered Peter's anguish in 1970 as he said to me, "My thinking is integral with my doing"—he had feared that he would not be able to think imaginatively about how to solve problems if he couldn't also get his hands on them. About this time, he was sometimes anxious that the stroke might have permanently affected his creative capacity. One day, as I saw him sitting with a pensive look on his face, I asked if he was having an idea. "No," he said sadly, "my thoughts are like little fish. They flash past—whisht, whisht—and I can't catch them." But the fish did get caught again as we lowered the drugs which controlled the blood pressure and the risk of seizures.

Early in 1972 a letter arrived informing Peter that the Queen proposed to make him a Companion of Honour. This is a civil Order, given for public and honourable service, and is bestowed at the choice of the Queen, to whom the recipient becomes a Companion. The investiture was to be held on 4 February in Buckingham Palace. The Queen received us in her drawing room. When she opened the box to show Peter the very pretty Order and spoke about its history, he was much moved—it would be an honour for a perfectly well man, and for one who had climbed back after being totally knocked from his perch this was a real moment of glory. I helped him to sit down, after he had received the Order, and the Queen firmly held the back of the chair for him, as Peter said afterwards, "To prevent me rolling backwards out of the Presence" on the well-oiled castors of the gilt chair.

As Peter became free from the side effects of the anti-seizure drugs, ideas came crowding back. He decided that we should "commit," as he called it, another book, a sort of biological dictionary, and that it would be called *From Aristotle to Zoos*, the capital letters of the first and last entries. He had heard that the ideal place to write a book is the Villa Serbelloni on the peninsula facing south at one end of Lake Como in Italy. He accordingly wrote to the Rockefeller Foundation in New York asking if we might spend three weeks there in September, and after a good deal of delay a date was arranged.

The Villa Serbelloni had been built in the fifteenth century by the Sforza family and had been rescued from disrepair when the last of the family married an American lady, Ella Wheeler, of great taste and wealth. She restored the tapestries, the furniture and the fine terraced gardens, and arranged that when she died the property should pass to the Rockefeller Foundation for the use of scholars. She also left sufficient money to retain the indoor staff of some thirty men and women and the outdoor staff of forty gardeners.

In September we flew to Milan, the nearest airport to the Villa Serbelloni. By now we had a routine at airports: we had a pre-ordered wheelchair at both ends of the journey, and Peter climbed the steps into the aircraft where necessary with only a little help from me. On one occasion one of the airline staff stood in front of Peter and asked me, "Can he walk?" as though he was inanimate. Peter didn't mind, being above such mistakes, but I did, and so might other wheelchair travellers. I took the stewardess on one side and asked her to remember in future that inability to walk was not incompatible with ability to think, and work, and hear. She reacted well and I felt better.

In Milan we were met by one of the drivers from the Villa Serbelloni, and within an hour of negotiating the hairpin bends along the lakeside road, we swept past the lodge gates of the estate and up the S-bends of the private road as it climbed the hill to the front porch of the Villa. The drive was long enough to allow the gardener who lived in the lodge to telephone the ideal host and hostess, Bill and Betsy Olson, who were waiting to welcome us at the front door.

Anyone lucky enough to be allowed to stay in the Villa as a scholar in residence came into the sort of ménage which rarely falls to a scholar's lot. We had a suite of rooms overlooking the lake on one side and the gardens on the other, and a balcony from which you could see the sun setting over the mountains. Because of Peter's difficulty in walking, we didn't go downstairs to breakfast; warm, crusty rolls, unsalted butter curls (no foil-wrapped portions here), coffee and black cherry jam were brought up to our room.

Peter worked at a table in the library in the mornings and as staff often passed quietly by the room, he could ask them to help if he needed anything. I could then go downhill through the terraces, which smelt of roses and warm box hedges, to a rock beside the lake, from which it was easy to slide into the cool water and swim along the shore.

During this visit we practised walking. At first, it was difficult for Peter to walk from the drawing room across the gravel on the terrace out to the table under the cedar tree, even though Franco, the head butler, was waiting there to serve drinks from a table. But we practised daily along the carpeted corridor outside our room, "right, and left, together with the stick," and soon graduated to a flight of shallow steps in the garden, taken with the left leg first. Once, as we reached the top, we heard gentle applause. Sir Karl Popper, another visiting scholar, had been watching us from the window of his room and had come down to help. One day he tried to help Peter walk on the flat terrace in front of the house. He came too close, in order to hear what Peter was saying, and caught his foot in Peter's stick. Peter fell flat on his back into a bed of ageratums and his head just missed the trunk of a pomegranate tree. Such an accident turns the stomach once it is over, and Karl was more shaken than Peter. I remember that Peter, lying in the flower bed, had first looked surprised and then laughed to relieve everyone's anxiety. For several days afterwards the impression his weight had made in the flower bed reminded me of what had happened, but it must have puzzled the gardeners.

Towards the end of the visit, Professor Willard van Quine, the distinguished American philosopher, came to stay as another scholar in residence. Normally wives did not stay at the Villa, so in introducing me Peter said apologetically, "She's my left leg, you know." Introducing Mrs. van Quine, who had come up from the hotel where she was staying to the Villa for tea, Professor van Quine replied, "And *she* is my left hemisphere." "I wish I'd said that," Peter replied, and I only just stopped myself from saying, "You will, Peter, you will."

Peter's walking improved so much during this visit that we began to play Ping-Pong together. The table stood in a damp grotto, glassed in on one side and built into the hillside, not too far from the house. If Peter had had full use of both hands and legs we would not have had so much fun; but I grumbled because I was the one who had to salvage all the wild balls from under the table, among ferns and out of the window. Peter spent a lot of time working systematically on the dictionary and enjoyed it each time he thought of a new biological term and a good way to describe it. Sometimes, but not so often, I thought of one and he was always delighted. He never made me feel the junior partner—as I was.

A few days before we left the Villa, Peter said that he wanted to come down to the shore to see where I swam, and then to climb back with me all the way to the top terrace. Young men, walking very fast, could do this uphill course in four to five minutes; I never managed less than seven. I thought the plan was probably not feasible, but for morale it was worth trying, providing we had help, concealed from Peter. It was arranged that a car should wait at two points on the climb where the S-bends of the road up to the Villa intersected the straight, uphill path through the orchards. The climb took us over half an hour, counting stops. The last part was up two flights of steps leading to the top terrace. Franco knew what was happening and became so excited that he left the drinks table and leant over the balustrade with Peter's favourite drink in his hand, calling out encouragement. No harm came from the exertion, and Peter was greatly pleased by his success—and by the progress he had made, not just in writing but in leading a more normal life.

The improvement in walking made a great difference to our lives. He felt more independent and I didn't have to walk quite so slowly beside him, but he still needed a rest in the middle of the day—and no wonder. Each time I took the heavy splint off his leg at night, I wondered how he could walk at all.

The splint prevented the left knee from bending back too far, but the metal hinge at the joint cut a small slice in the left trouser leg, spoiling every good suit. Peter refused to wear anything but a sober suit, enlivened by ties which Jerry Lawrence (the naval doctor friend who had got us off the *QE2*) sent from New York, or his family bought him for birthdays. Fortunately we found a reasonably priced tailor (God bless the firm of Charkhams) who sent a Mr. Newman to the house to design suits which avoided the cutting hinge of the splint and provided the many pockets Peter insisted on. Mr. Newman came to admire him enormously and took a lot of trouble. He was a great encourager, too, noticing any improvement that had been made between his visits.

Every bedtime Peter carried out a nightly ritual of laying out the contents of many pockets—keys, glasses, wallet, pen, tiny note pad and cotton handkerchief (he hated even strong paper handkerchiefs). Most people spend frustrating minutes every day chasing missing property. Because he kept so many things in his suit, Peter rarely did. When I regularly mislaid the car or house key, I think it gave him satisfaction to be able to say, as I turned everything upside down in looking for it, "Here, don't worry— have mine."

His working day was now almost back to normal but with less

pressure—and with a sleep in a reclining chair after lunch in his office. His colleagues looked after him in the laboratory in every possible way. Heinz Wolff, head of Bioengineering at the Clinical Research Centre, designed and maintained an electric wheelchair in which Peter learnt to speed down the passages, bang through the double swing doors, and enter lifts backwards at top speed, to the alarm of those in it who did not already know from experience what was happening.

The work he and his team were doing was in due course routinely inspected by a group from the Medical Research Council. The group reported that there were enough ideas in it to last the team for several years, and Peter was greatly pleased.

At home a mixture of car, wheelchair and walking stick allowed us to go out for entertainment when we felt like it. Twice a week one of a rota of girls would come in after supper, to stay the night and give me the chance of long night's sleep. At first, they could not understand how someone of my size could help someone of Peter's to hoist himself up or down from a chair, but they soon discovered that the performance was based on cunning, not on strength, and learnt how to do it themselves.

By now, Peter's illness and recovery were pretty well known to his friends and colleagues, and they did not forget to think of ways to interest him. The Director of the army research station at Porton not only invited us to lunch but arranged for us to be flown by helicopter from the Royal Air Force base at Northolt, just outside London. As I drove our car alongside the waiting helicopter, there was an impressive display of saluting. The officer in charge suggested that I should "snap out a few orders" because getting a six-foot-four-inch hemiplegic distinguished scientist up into a helicopter had not, he said, been part of his training. It hadn't been part of mine either, but with two strong sergeants to do the lifting, it wasn't difficult. Peter was soon strapped in and we took off with a rattling whirlwind of noise. From our height the

pattern of the countryside looked like a large-scale map and we
flew so low that the racket of our flight scared the birds out of the
hedgerows.

Porton was built in the middle of Salisbury Plain, and during
the war part of the research there was on chemical warfare. I don't
know what Peter discussed with his friend the Director because I
was invited to drive in the game warden's jeep to visit a pair of
Great Bustards, large rare birds, related to turkeys. They had been
installed in a huge area of rough grass, protected by a wire fence,
by the British Bustard Society, to save them from the threat of
extinction. Two greater contrasts of intention could hardly have
existed beside each other—Porton Down for research into chemical warfare and a safe breeding ground for Great Bustards.

On 28 May 1972, Peter had a three-minute seizure early in the
morning for no discernable reason. By this time neither of us
reacted as though the end of the world was approaching, but the
sight of someone out of control was always awful all the same.
After an attack I gave him a quarter of a Mogadon at night, and we
went early to bed and carried on as usual the next day.

Jacques Monod, the French biologist and 1965 Nobel Laureate,
came to visit a few days later and his delight at Peter's progress
encouraged us both. They talked as old scientific friends talk when
they haven't seen each other for a while, and he and Peter discussed the theme of Monod's book *Chance and Necessity* for
nearly an hour. The BBC recorded their conversation for Radio 3
in a programme called "The New Biology."

Monod's *Chance and Necessity* had caused a sensation, not
just because of its content but because of the distinction of its
author. In 1965 he had won the Nobel Prize for his discovery of
the biological function of the substance DNA, which encodes
within it the instructions for reproduction. The essence of Monod's
opinion was that there is no scientific authority for believing that
life has a purpose, or is going anywhere . . . and that all such

beliefs are part of "a disgusting farrago of animistic Judaeo-Christian religiosity, scientistic progressivism and belief in the rights of man." After introducing Jacques's discovery of the function of genetic regulation, one of the most crucial discoveries of the twentieth century, Peter referred to the "disgusting farrago" passage and said, "Now I don't believe that you wrote the book in order to bring these dismal tidings to anybody. What *was* the motive?" Monod replied that a large part of his reason for writing was "to try and clarify my own mind as to the relationship between the values I respect and the field in which I happen to have been working." He was not, he said, attacking the values themselves, as some people mistakenly believed.

Monod went on to one passage which he had cut from his book. In this passage he imagined that Martians had landed their space ship on a Greek island near some windmills, in order to study which of the objects they saw on earth were artefacts and which natural objects. When a big discussion arose as to whether the mills were serving the men or the men the mills, the Martians decided to have a symposium, calling in all the authorities. "Naturally," Monod said to Peter, "you were there, and so was Francis Crick."

Peter laughed, "How typical of them that they should hold a symposium to try and resolve the matter. I'm sorry you cut that passage out."

During the rest of the interview they discussed the theory of ageing, progress in medical biology, Karl Popper's view of the exploratory process of science, the nature of truth, evolution, Chomsky's theory of language and the nature of value judgements. It was a dazzling discussion and it elated me: nothing could have better illustrated Peter's astonishing recovery.

All through 1971 Barbara Ward had been preparing her marvellous book *Only One Earth* for the United Nations Conference in Stockholm on Man and His Environment. She and I had been

scholars at Somerville together but we had lost touch during her
career as an economist. Now, thirty years later, we had a common
concern for the fate of the environment; Barbara already had one
hundred consultants of many different nationalities advising on
the scientific aspects of the book. In addition she invited Peter to
check the biology and me to approve the section on population. In
exchange for this small contribution, she arranged that we went as
guests to Stockholm to stay in the Grand Hotel. As Peter limped
into the hotel the doorman stepped forward and greeted us by
name—he had remembered him from the Nobel ceremony twelve
years earlier.

I went to the meetings and Peter stayed in the hotel to read the
papers prepared by each of the 116 nations attending. Later he
wrote a beautiful review of Barbara's book *Only One Earth* under
the title "House in Order," in which he contrasted her outlook with
John Maddox's thinking in his book *The Doomsday Syndrome*.
The review ended: "It is the great strength of Barbara Ward's text
that she argues so cogently for keeping our house in order, and it
is the weakness of Maddox's that he does not seem clearly enough
to realise that there is anything very serious to worry about."*
There is no doubt now about which outlook was wiser.

By now Peter's reputation as a writer brought him more invitations to speak on general subjects than he could manage. He
designed a formula for refusing politely: "I have made it a practice
not to accept more than one invitation each month, and I regret
that . . ." He did however accept an invitation from IBM's Centre
at Rochester in New York State. It provided every inducement and
made allowance for his physical handicaps. So we flew to New
York at the end of 1972 and were met at Kennedy Airport by one
of IBM's staff, Dr. Benoit Mandlebrot, sometimes known as the
Wizard of Fractals. I had never heard of fractals, but Peter had,

---

*Quoted in *Pluto's Republic* (London: Oxford University Press, 1984), p. 286.

and as Dr. Mandlebrot drove us towards Rochester I listened with delight to a mathematical conversation I couldn't understand. Peter's memory was entirely up to it and they laughed and talked as equals.

His role at IBM was not to discuss mathematics, but to infuse into the computer world ideas and problems from his world of medical science, in case a strict diet of computer science might turn all these extremely clever Jacks into dull boys. During the discussions after his talk I noticed that while Peter had sparkled with Dr. Mandlebrot, it was very difficult for him to manage cross talk with a big, bright group. Partly he was tired and partly he could not see all of them; the left side of the circle they were sitting in, for him, did not exist. Some of the questions were ones that didn't stimulate him—on the lines of isn't-too-much-knowledge-dangerous, weren't-we-all-getting-too-soft-in-our-controlled-environments, and so on. Here, I knew what Peter thought, and when he turned to ask what my opinion was, I filled in. I don't think the visit gave them any idea of Peter's stature, but it was an extremely interesting one, and everybody was very considerate.

Before his stroke in 1969, Peter had been appointed as a scientific consultant at the Sloan-Kettering Cancer Center in New York. After his illness his American colleagues took a very positive view of whether or not he should continue coming over to New York for consultations. Of course he should, and they couldn't do without him, was their attitude, and it was a tonic for Peter, for which I am forever grateful. The consultants met twice a year. The Director, then Dr. Robert Good, presided, while members of the scientific staff presented reports on current research and on future proposals which were then generally discussed. The company was congenial, the research interesting and the hospitality excellent, so we much looked forward to these meetings. On one of them, during a visit to inspect laboratory work, one research worker demonstrated that a skin graft from one mouse to another had taken after having been cultured for some time outside the donor's body. At the end of the visit Peter mentioned to me that he had sensed a curious atmosphere in this laboratory, and an unease when he asked questions. He claimed that a rabbit which was supposed to have received a corneal graft into the eye had looked at him with a "candid gaze" as though no operation had touched it. Neither of us thought much more about what the rabbit's expression signified or what the atmosphere meant, until the scandal of the "painted mouse" spread out of the labs and into the newspapers, television and magazines. The researcher, Dr. Summerlin, had inked the shape of a black graft in the fur of the white mouse and had claimed to be able to do what no one else had found possible—to transplant skin successfully from one strain of mouse to another.

Summerlin was called a blackguard, a cheat and a liar, his early background was investigated and he was reported to have begun cheating at school. He was suspended from the laboratory and advised to seek psychiatric help. Of all the explanations of what had happened, Peter's was the most charitable. Summerlin, he said, genuinely believed that his experiments were succeeding— but he had been tempted to fake success before it had arrived, to show Dr. Good what progress he was making. He titivated the graft and was, unfortunately, given approval too easily. He needed success and so did the hospital, to attract more money for research.

In the summer of the Watergate scandal an invitation arrived from the Aspen Institute for the Humanities in Colorado. Peter was asked to be a sort of guru in residence at the Institute, to give one lecture and to take part in seminars for business people. The seminars were run by scholars from the arts, theatre, literature and science, and after a short presentation, discussion was open to the audience. Besides Peter, among the other "gurus" were Peter Brook and Herman Wouk. In August we flew to Denver, Colorado. There we changed into the very small plane which makes the run to Aspen over the Rocky Mountains. The flight was alarming. As we flew very low along a narrow valley, I watched forked lightning flashing out of the thunderclouds on both sides of the plane and hoped it might strike the mountains instead of us. I was glad that Peter's eyesight only allowed him to see out of the windows on the right side.

The air at Aspen was slightly rarefied and we were warned that we might feel a little breathless until we had adapted. We spent the first day quietly in a very pleasant small guest house, built on the banks of a tumbling stream. Chipmunks came out from their burrows under big rocks and entertained us with their mercurial agility as we fed them with breakfast crumbs. After two days Peter gave a lecture on science and literature; he wasn't tired after it, and we began to enjoy taking part in the seminars and discussions.

The day after Peter had given his lecture we tried taking a walk of about 100 yards from our house, along a path through the meadow which led to the conference buildings. Soon Peter's hand got very tired as it pressed heavily down on his walking stick and he needed to rest. I helped him to lean against one of the huge boulders beside the path and we paused before starting to walk back to the house.

As I looked around, I was surprised to see, a long way down the field path, what looked like a man riding a bicycle with folded arms. How unlikely, in this centre for the humanities, I thought. But it was, and as the man passed our rock, he called out cheerfully, "Don't you just *hate* a show-off?'' and then, almost immediately recognising Peter, he jumped off his bicycle and greeted us. It was Herman Wouk. He walked back to the house with us and we began conversations and another of the friendships which has grown steadily ever since.

In the following years Peter and he played chess by post, but Peter was an impatient chess player and often found the posts too slow. Our paths crossed at intervals and every meeting was full of spirit and amusement. On one occasion, twelve years later, when

Peter was in hospital, Herman and his wife Sarah invited me to dine with them at Claridges Hotel in London, assuming that the difficulty of getting Peter out of hospital and into the restaurant would be too great. But I thought I could manage, so I rang up to warn the head porter at the hotel to be ready, got Peter out of hospital and into a wheelchair and then into the car and out into the wheelchair again, and up the front steps of Claridges. The surprise for Herman was worth the effort. He was so delighted he wanted to punch Peter in the "you old son of a gun" way men do. The expedition was a landmark in Peter's recovery. Eating an elegant dish of fish at table, with linen napkins, talking to Herman and Sarah, was very different from sitting up in a hospital bed with supper on a tray, listening to the hushed conversations of other people's relatives.

The success of the Aspen expedition increased our confidence about travelling, so when Professor Walter Brendl, a surgeon who knew Peter's work, invited us to join a conference of young immunologists and surgeons in Kitzbühel I was delighted and Peter was quite keen. He had never been to Austria in winter and I had always wanted him to see the beauty of a snow-covered landscape in sunshine. He had consistently vetoed skiing—breaking one of his long legs would be too time-consuming, he thought.

The company Walter Brendl brought to the very comfortable Tennerhof Gasthaus in Kitzbühel was bright and lively. The story about how he selected his graduate students was plausible. They had to be intelligent, of course, but besides that it was almost obligatory to have either a good singing voice or a marked talent for skiing.

Our stay began well: a lady approached Peter as we came into the hall of the Gasthaus, and seeing his arm in a sling, asked him sympathetically on which Piste he had had his accident. Throughout his strokes and seizure he always looked well, but to be taken for an athlete at this stage was a big encouragement.

At this conference nobody worked until after lunch but I believe that as much useful work was achieved as if they had been going all day. Everyone spent the morning skiing: some of the immunologists were members of the German ski team. They were also good teachers and I enjoyed myself enormously.

By the time we got back to London we had a feeling that we were leading an almost normal life, in spite of the handicaps. But one day Peter had not arrived home by seven o'clock. He had been driven down to Kent on a visit to the Wellcome Laboratories and was due back at six. As he invariably liked to have supper ready by seven my old dread of another stroke revived. At last the telephone rang and a man who introduced himself as a doctor said confidently, "Your husband has had another stroke and has been taken to University College Hospital."

I think it is impossible to prepare for such news. It may be like being shot. The only mercy is a temporary numbness and a sense of disbelief. I warned myself to drive carefully, but got to the hospital very quickly. Someone told me I couldn't go into the room where Peter was, but of course I did, and found him alone and miserable. As soon as I saw him I was sure he had had a small seizure and not a stroke. His relief at my arrival was touching: I know he was casting me in the role of Beethoven's Fidelio, who rescues her husband from a dark dungeon. I was very angry with the doctor who had telephoned me, but it was Dr. Michael Kremer who really sorted him out as he arrived to see Peter. "And *what* reason have you for supposing that Sir Peter has had a stroke?" I heard him ask, so coldly that I felt almost sorry for the young man.

Peter stayed the night in the hospital, but I drove him home the next day, we pulled ourselves together and life went on normally. The next day he began reading and preparing for the presentation of one of a series of Doubleday lectures at the Smithsonian Institute in Washington.

There was a formal dinner in the Smithsonian before the lecture, and as the coffee was being served the sound of many feet on stone floors and many voices greeting each other showed that a large audience was arriving. Before they had finished arriving, the organiser realised that the lecture room would not hold them all. The museum carpenters were called to improvise a raised platform so that Peter could be seen while lecturing right in the middle of one of the exhibition halls, underneath a huge statue of George Washington. For once he got his notes thoroughly mixed—easily done if you have only half the normal eyesight. In the middle of the lecture he stopped suddenly and said, quite unflustered, "I seem to have lost my way in the scenario. Jeanie, where are you?" I climbed onto the platform and sorted out the notes. As I got down, Peter smiled at the audience and said, "I see what she means; page 4 comes *after* page 3." He couldn't have done better. The audience was delighted and before he could go on he had to wait for the laughter to die down.

March, back in England, brought two unpleasant setbacks; the epididymal cyst needed draining again and there was another seizure—but it was the last of the series of thirteen. The change in the daily pattern of life did not vary noticeably and Peter treated his handicaps with a brave indifference. He was driven to the Clinical Research Centre every day, continued writing, going to conferences and planning research. We had evenings at Covent Garden or at the theatre or with friends and he even managed dinner with Margaret Thatcher, the Prime Minister. All I can remember him saying about that was "I didn't get a word in"—but he wasn't complaining.

We were lucky that Caroline, Charles and Loulie often came for a family supper at weekends. Loulie had now come back from Chicago with her husband, Len, whom she had helped through medical school. Until we bought a small house for them, they and their two children—Benjamin, aged seven and Siiri aged one—lived with us at Mount Vernon House. Peter needed help with

dressing and the children were imaginative and gentle in helping
him to find things. His feet were size 13 and their great shape
fascinated them. They powdered each foot before the socks went
on, so diligently that Peter called them his "powder monkeys."

Peter gained strength gradually but his tempo had to be much
slower than before the stroke. He was still enchanted by ideas—
he called them "imaginative forays into the world of hy-
potheses"—but he became much easier to know and appreciated
ordinary people for non-intellectual qualities he might not have
noticed before. He took pains to be especially nice to strangers
who sometimes became involved in helping us in or out of the car.
If an American gave him a powerful lift, he would say apprecia-
tively, "You must have played fullback for Notre Dame"; they
liked the compliment and he enjoyed delivering it. The English
compliment was on the lines that the strong man must be "a great
Christian gentleman," spoken as if it was in capital letters, and this
immediately relaxed any of the embarrassment sometimes produced by handicaps.

ELEVEN

Moves and Travels,
1974-1980

IN 1975 WE LEFT Mount Vernon House. When I looked up Peter's contract with the Medical Research Council, I found that the house was ours only while Peter was working as their employee. I could not be sure how long he might be able to go on working, and as we could not reasonably expect to live in the house if he were not, I began house-hunting.

Loulie had become a very practical young woman, and having decided—after a third beautiful child called Peter—that she had married the wrong man, she developed a successful mail-order business to help support her family and Len went back to America. She helped me hunt and we soon found a very pretty terrace house in Downshire Hill. The terrace runs down to Hampstead Heath at its east end and up to the village at the other. The houses were built about 1834 from bricks made from local clay and each has long gardens at the back where there had been orchards of pear and apple trees.

In spring the windows look out onto clouds of white blossom. At the end of summer when the pear trees are loaded with small unripe pears, flocks of starlings move in to eat the fruit. Our pear tree becomes full of moving black wings, the sound of fluttering and clucking and pecking, and by the time the birds leave, only the fruit stalks are left. It fascinates me that the starlings can safely cope with a once a year diet of bullet-hard pears.

The worst part of moving was looking after the books. By now we had about 1,500, catalogued and in order on the shelves. I paid the movers extra to keep the books on each shelf as they were arranged; this shouldn't have been difficult because the shelves were labelled and had already been taken from Mount Vernon and put up in Downshire Hill. I told Peter not to worry about the books—I had "fixed" the movers. The men assured me they were used to moving whole libraries and I believed them—until I started putting the books back on their shelves in the new house. They could not have done a better job if I had paid them to randomise the titles.

When we had moved from Birmingham to London in 1952, Peter was only forty-seven and he was extremely energetic. His maxim about all the things that needed doing was "Do it now." If you didn't, he had noticed, it would probably never get done. He assembled a tool box and spent all his weekend time wiring up lamps, fixing up mirrors, pictures and towel rails, as capably as any odd job man. Inevitably the children used to borrow the tools, usually for purposes for which they were not meant. When a tool was returned—as it sometimes was—the end of the screwdriver might be covered in rapid glue or the blades of the saw bent and minus several teeth. Peter would be exasperated and would threaten, mock-seriously, "Just *wait* till you have a tool box and children. I shall bribe them to hide and damage every tool, regularly and systematically."

Peter hated disorder. In his world every tool, book or utensil had to be put back in its place at the end of its use. Displacement or mess meant more work and less time for what he wanted to do next.

After Peter's stroke I had to inherit the tool box; but even with two hands I was slower than he had been at mending fuses and putting new plugs on lamps, and for any carpentry or alteration I needed help. A friend recommended a Jamaican builder and carpenter, Mr. Ivan Price. Mr. Price could do almost any job except estimate its cost. He would simply say, "Whateffer you tink, Leddy Medwar." What I thought was an estimate based on hours and materials, and on this basis Mr. Price became an invaluable help.

The house in Downshire Hill is arranged on four floors; on the garden level were two bed sitting rooms, a small bathroom and a passage that opened into an area from which iron steps led to the front garden, and the street. On the next floor the front door opened into a small lobby for coats, leading into a dining room; beyond that was the kitchen, which looked out onto the pear trees in the long garden. On the floor above was the sitting room, at the front of the house, and the book-lined study at the back. On the top floor, above this, we had our bathroom and bedroom, both carpeted and lined with cupboards. I found a partners desk for the study, under which Peter's high knees could fit, and we sat on either side of it, each with a set of drawers and a view over the garden. A year later, when we were sitting and writing opposite each other at the desk, Peter stopped writing, looked up and said, "This is just how I hoped it would be when we began." That was now thirty-eight years ago.

In the summer of the Queen's Silver Jubilee, Peter had a letter from Victor Rothschild introducing a brilliant American photographer, Bernard Schwartz, who had come to England with his wife Ronny in order to photograph people with "Outstanding Features." Each sitter was to be given a large framed photograph of themselves, which looked deceptively like an oil painting. Bern and Ronny planned to sell prints of the portraits at an exhibition in Colnaghi's Gallery and to give the proceeds to the Queen's Silver Jubilee Fund. I found this idea for raising funds surprising, because the sitters, though very distinguished, were not household names, though perhaps Clare Francis, who sailed single-handed round the world, Lord Rothschild, Geraint Evans the opera singer, Angela Rippon the TV news reader, and Lester Piggott the famous jockey were. So who would buy? Anyway, excellent photographs were taken and exhibited and the sale raised £11,000; everyone was pleased. Later Ronny Schwartz organised the portraits into a book and raised another £10,000 for the Covent Garden Opera Fund.

One day she rang me to exchange news. She and Bern had been invited to Buckingham Palace for dinner. The Israeli general Moshe Dayan was delighted with his portrait, and the new Pope wanted Bern to come to Rome in order to photograph him in the Vatican. "Where do we go from here?" Ronny asked ironically. I suggested that Europe was probably as full of Outstanding Features as England. Then her voice changed from its normal confident tone. "There's just one other thing," she said. "Bern has a pain." What she described was clearly not a one-aspirin pain, so I suggested doctors whom she should consult. The diagnosis was very bad: it was cancer of the pancreas. Ronny wanted to assemble all available experts in their home in San Diego. I persuaded her, after taking advice, that this expensive exercise could not help Bern. Instead, he and she bravely accepted that he had not long to live and concentrated on the quality of the time left. When they got home, Ronny and I corresponded and in one of her letters she wrote that they "were at peace." I was very moved by their dignity and courage and adaptability—their lives had plummeted from international acclaim to Bern's death within a single year—and I remembered it when we had our difficulties.

By March 1978, Peter's cyst became uncomfortable and needed draining again. He had it done the day before we were due to leave for the scientific consultants' meeting in New York. This time there were after-effects. Halfway over the Atlantic he began to feel wretched. Soon he was shivering and we knew that he had started an infection. The journey seemed endless. At Kennedy Airport one of the Sloan-Kettering drivers who knew us was waiting and he drove us as fast as he could to Abby Aldrich Hall where a room had been arranged for us. I got Peter into bed and rang the Sloan-Kettering Hospital, on York Avenue just opposite, to ask for help. As usual Peter was half stoical and half tending to pooh-pooh the idea that there was anything much the matter. Fortunately Dr. Whitmore the surgeon who came over from the hospital was both kind and very firm; in spite of the protests, he summoned a wheelchair and an intern and we pushed the shivering, blanketed Peter across the traffic of York Avenue and into the hospital. There Dr. Whitmore dealt with the problem under local anaesthetic. This was at Peter's request, and was on condition that he might have morphine after the operation.

The next day I was sitting beside his bed in the hospital with Professor Richard Beard, a friend from England, when a nurse came in bearing a syringe. "Is it my promised morphine?" Peter asked. It wasn't. Richard tactfully intervened, and she went away to change the prescription. After the injection Peter began smiling. "From now on," he murmured, "it's the poppy and the grape for me." He slept and rested for a day or two and recovered so quickly that he was able to give his lecture in the Abby Aldrich Hall as it had been scheduled. Those of the audience who knew that he had just come from an operation in hospital greeted him with admiring amazement.

His lecture on the story of the discovery of tolerance, from the cattle twins to Supermice, went smoothly. Afterward, we much enjoyed a small dinner for colleagues in the library of the Abby Aldrich. The next day we flew to Hawaii to stay with Eugene and Evelyn Lance. Eugene had left the Clinical Research Centre in 1977 announcing that, as he had already experienced the cream of scientific life, he was now off to sample the fleshpots, supported by an orthopaedic practice, in Honolulu. Some people pictured the Lances in a pastoral setting of grass skirts and plangent local music; but Evelyn, a lawyer and musicologist, retorted that whereas in Pinner, Middlesex, on the outskirts of London it had been a problem to find one friend with a harpsichord, in Hawaii it was easy to find four.

The Lances' house is built on a hillside overlooking the bay of Honolulu; they could not have looked after us better—they even moved out of their own big bedroom. Eugene left early morning for his orthopaedic practice and Evelyn for her sessions as a judge in the marital court. She had stocked the refrigerator with everything needed, so we had the house to ourselves, played their large collection of operatic recordings and practised gentle walks along the wide verandah in the sunshine.

Peter gave a lecture a few days after we arrived. He wasn't in very good form this time and I felt anxious that it might not have earned our keep. Eugene reproved me. "People don't expect Peter to perform as he did," he said; "what they honour is the work he has done and his courage in proceeding." The rest of the visit was idyllic—I could float in the swimming pool in their garden, and from it look up at Peter lying in a comfortable chair on the verandah. In the evening the Lances either took us to excellent restaurants or we ate at home, with wine chosen by Eugene to please Peter. One weekend they took us to stay in a hotel built on the lip of the volcano that rumbles away on the largest of the Hawaiian Islands. I loved this and the subsequent tour of the island and on

the drive home I thanked Eugene for the sightseeing. He laughed—
well, yes, he supposed it was good of him, because he wasn't
really interested. "Now, you, Peter," he said, "you'd also much
rather be at home in our house with music and a drink, wouldn't
you?" Peter reluctantly agreed. Gene shouted with joy and called
Peter a man after his own heart.

This visit to Hawaii shortened our winter. When we got home
Peter began to plan for the high point of his summer: the June
weekend test match at Lord's cricket ground. We used to invite
friends to arrive at our house at about ten on the Saturday morning.
On arrival they were offered a mixture called Buck's Fizz—half
fresh orange juice and half champagne. This was drunk while
listening to an old recording of Dame Clara Butt, the Australian
contralto, singing "Land of Hope and Glory." I don't know why
Peter invented this ritual but it amused him greatly. After Buck's
Fizz, twelve of us then drove in three cars to park as near as
possible to Lords; quite a feat, because from early in the day every
foot of every road near the cricket ground was packed with cars,
and the pavements crowded with people making their way to Lords.
Their faces wore expressions of content; they had tickets and were
anticipating the joys of watching a game in which anything can
happen at almost any time. A fast bowler can bowl at 90 miles an
hour at the batsman. The ball is made of leather, stretched and
sewn over an inside of hard wood, and it can and does occasionally
fracture a bone. Slow bowlers can make the ball describe bends in
the air to confuse the batsman, so to the initiated, the game is never
dull; so much depends on morale and luck as well as skill.

To reach the seats that Peter had booked early in the year, we
had to walk along concrete paths under the raked and covered
stands and then climb up two flights of stone steps. We always
dreamt that the sun would be out and the players in white flannels
would show up above their dark shadows on the green grass; but it
often rained and that stopped play, or the light was bad and that

stopped it too. In spite of this, Peter's pleasure in the day was infectious and we all felt happy. For each of us I packed a bag containing a small crusty pork pie, a hard-boiled egg, a cheese sandwich, a tomato, and a slice of fruit cake, all drunk with plenty of beer. Charles, now thirty-seven, had distinguished himself at cricket while at Westminster School and he always came, later on with his wife Caroline. He, David Pyke and Leslie Brent were regulars in the party, and they helped Peter up the stairs and into a seat in the stands. The journalist Katherine Whitehorn brought fruit and dragged her husband Gavin Lyall along, but in the end he liked it too. Our three medical friends, James Gowans, David, and Robert Sells, sometimes hadn't met for a year and if there were any longueurs in the game they had plenty of medical gossip to exchange. The trouble about cricket is that sometimes the best catch of the match is taken while you are not looking. In one of her articles for the *Observer* Katherine once toyed with the idea that there might be some causal connection.

Later on that summer we did what we had wanted to do for the last thirty years: we went to Bayreuth for a whole week of Wagner's *Ring* cycle. Bernard Levin—who knows everything about opera and especially Wagner—told Peter that there was only one place to stay, the Post Hotel in Pegnitz. The Post Hotel has been run by the Pflaum family for four hundred years, and during this time they have learnt a great deal about pleasing guests. Bernard said that when he had arrived, late and tired, Herr Pflaum was waiting up to welcome him. In his room was fruit, a chilled bottle of wine, and what the first-class menu on some airlines call "Amuses bouches"—only these delicacies really did amuse the bouche.

We flew first to Freiburg and stayed with Otto Westphal and his wife Uschi. We had met for the first time at a conference in Brussels where he and Peter were advisers to Christian de Duves, the Director of the great Institute for Cellular Pathology. Otto had watched how Peter and I were managing; I think he thought we needed a holiday. He said to me, "I've just won rather a large prize. Now I know what we'll do with it. We'll have a trip together from Freiburg down to Lucerne." And so it was arranged.

After a day's rest with them, they packed us into their big car and took us touring, through the dark evergreens of the Black Forest, stopping at high-up village inns for simple good food and cool white wine, and then down to the shining levels of Lake Lucerne. There we stayed as Otto's guests in a splendid hotel.

We finished the tour at the Pflaums' Post Hotel in Pegnitz. Everything in the hotel smelt right. At the front door geraniums, marguerites and lobelias spilled out of big tubs; they were watered and fed every day and they looked as flowers do in seed catalogues. The covers of the eiderdowns had probably been dried in the sun, the floors were polished but not slippery, and the food and service were excellent.

The Westphals preferred chamber music to Wagner, so they left that pleasure to us and drove back to Freiburg. In the early evening a small bus belonging to the hotel took us into Bayreuth in good time for the performance and brought us back for a late supper in the hotel restaurant. One evening as we were finishing our soup, Peter looked up sharply as two men and two women came in to dine. "My God," he said, "it's Gwyneth Jones"—she had been singing Brunnhilde a few hours earlier. I said I thought it couldn't be because she was chattering in German without the slightest accent, but the next night the same party returned and this time I saw Peter was right. I knew he was longing to meet Gwyneth. He remembered that she had married a Swiss business man called Till Haberfeld. I asked the waiter for some paper and an envelope and sent a message over to their table: "My husband is longing to congratulate your wife. It is difficult for him to stand. He would appreciate it very much if you could pass our table as you go out." We watched the effect of this note. Gwyneth and Till and their companions scanned the restaurant for the likely writers.

They decided, probably by elimination, that it was us, then, long before they had finished, Till brought Gwyneth over to sit by Peter and talk to us.

Gwyneth is the sort of girl success does not spoil. After a tremendous success she can laugh and say, "Not bad for a girl from Pontypool,* eh?" She is open, affectionate, and understanding, and Till knows well how to orchestrate their separate and joint lives. We started a friendship that evening which gives constant pleasure. Sometimes we have met in a plane going to New York, sometimes they come home to dinner with us, and sometimes we have a late dinner with them after the opera. I had imagined that an opera singer would be tired after a performance and would want to go to bed. Not Gwyneth. Her mood remains high, she looks radiant, feels wonderful and eats heartily.

The first time she and Till dined with us at home, I cooked a steak and kidney pie. We also invited Shirley Conran, a successful journalist, three German friends, and a musical neurologist, and it was a good party. When I cleared away the plates it was Gwyneth, the diva, who jumped up to help carry them into the kitchen.

The second time we went to Bayreuth, the Haberfelds invited us to have dinner with them after the opera. At this time, it wasn't difficult to extract Peter from the car and up onto his feet—but you had to know where to place your weight. Whenever Gwyneth met Peter, she took on the role of a Valkyrie: removing a fallen hero from the battlefield and up to the joys of Valhalla, as in the opera. She caught hold of his arm and, being a strong girl, she pulled hard upwards. I heard the dreaded rip-rip noise of stitches tearing, and as she got Peter on his feet I could see white shirt sleeve through the torn armhole. Gwyneth reacted with her normal humour and serenity. She looked at the damage, smiled, and said, "Never mind. I'm sure Jean is *very* good at mending."

* Her small home town in Wales.

Not long after we came home from Pegnitz, the mail brought Peter one of the nicest benefactions he ever earned. The Alfred Sloan Foundation commissioned him to write a book, to be one of a series from different authors each designed to open windows into the world of the scientist through which laymen might understand its importance, its threats and glories, and how to take an intelligent interest in its applications. The commission was generously funded, and quite enough for long and comfortable travelling. We decided to visit Peter's sister in Cape Province, South Africa, where she and her surgeon husband Sir Ian McAdam had built a house and made a farm on land Ian had bought twenty-five years before. Pam warned us that even young people got off the plane in Johannesburg in a state of exhaustion, but Peter felt exhilarated by the whole prospect. He had the idea of the book he was going to write in outline in his head and looked forward to starting.

In this mood and once on board the plane to Johannesburg, he celebrated with one too many cocktails, before dinner, a long-delayed dinner. He felt and was very sick, but in spite of this and the long journey, as we walked from the plane towards where Pam and Ian were waiting for us at Port Elizabeth, he managed to perform his favourite trick—throwing up his walking stick to turn a circle in the air and return to his hand. We were tired, though, and slept very late next day. We woke to a cloudless sky, brilliant sunshine, and Pam, bearing a welcome breakfast.

In the twenty-five years before building the house we were in, Ian McAdam had built up the surgery department at Makere Hospital in Uganda to a very high level, training young surgeons to his standards without concern for the colour of their skin. When the tyrant Iddi Amin came to power this was Ian's undoing, for Amin was as bad and cruel as Hitler about so-called race. Soon the Asians who used to bring the oxygen cylinders to the hospital were found in the hospital grounds with their throats cut, and the newspapers, radio and television ran the headline "Sir Ian McAdam

Spreads Political Gonorrhoea." Ian and Pam packed the best of their possessions into a camping car, bought two train tickets and got out of Uganda into Zimbabwe just before the worst of the bloodbaths.

There was no shortage of prospects for Ian. He was offered jobs with the National Health Service in England and the National Institutes of Health in Bethesda in the States. But after the responsibilities he had taken, the proposals didn't really appeal. What he wanted was to make two blades of grass grow where only one had grown before, and to do it with Pam and in sunshine.

This intention prospered, and by the time we were in a position to visit them in Plettenberg Bay, they had built a beautiful house, a guest house, a garden, and two lakes; they farmed sheep, cattle, ducks, and planted strawberry fields on land bounded by a long line of trees and a view over the mountains and the Indian Ocean. Pam said that, except for apartheid, it was like a millionaire's paradise; but there was apartheid. The McAdams' nearest neighbour was a lawyer who lived ten miles away. This man had been brave enough to testify that the police had beaten up a black man while he was in their custody. Thereafter a police van would drive threateningly round their house at night and his children were stopped and frightened on their way to school.

We stayed for a perfect three weeks. Pam and Ian were great company, the sun shone, I could help in the garden and swim at Plettenberg Bay. There the rollers of the Indian Ocean curled gently onto the superb sandy shore. Peter couldn't dress correctly for an ocean dip—he still had his massive leg splint on, he walked with a stick and needed a sun hat. When we got down to the water's edge he discarded the paraphernalia, sat down with difficulty on the sand and let the ripples cool his legs; but Pam and I had to watch out—anything much bigger than a ripple would bowl him sideways, and one almost did.

In the mornings Peter worked hard on the book which had

brought us there. It was called *Advice to a Young Scientist,* and it
streamed fluently out of his head and into his small hand-held tape
recorder. I thought it was going to be good, because recording
sessions were often punctuated by shouts of laughter which I could
hear from the room in which I was writing a small book, *Lifeclass.*
Peter slept in the afternoons and dictated again after tea. Pam is a
generous and superb cook, and in the evening we drank good local
wine by a wood fire.

Around 6:00 p.m. Ian came home from Knysna, the hospital a
few miles down the coast where he had intended to do part-time
surgery; but surgeons of his quality had not been known there
before he came, and he was soon working full time for half pay.
At dinner he told us interesting and sometimes awful stories. Once
he described how a man had been brought to him impaled through
the chest with the shaft of a large cart. I asked Ian what he had
done. "Got the carpenter to saw it off and then got to work," he
said. "And what happened to the man?" "Oh," Ian answered, "he
was as right as rain in a week." A lot of his time was taken up
repairing wounds from knife fights. On pay day it had been traditional for the work force to drink heavily—a legacy from the
wicked old habit of paying part of the workers' wages in drink.
These were no friendly punch-ups between different tribes; they
knifed each other murderously, usually in the guts.

Sometimes I helped Pam by picking strawberries for market.
She sold them locally and put the money into a Going Home Fund.
She suggested that we might promote sales by labelling our baskets
as "Picked by Real Ladies." That might not have been so comic,
either; after all, the black waiters in a big hotel at Plettenberg Bay
were dressed as eighteenth-century English sailors, with pigtails.

We hated to leave Pam and Ian, the comfortable life and the
sunshine—it could be a long time before we would meet again—
and we felt rather depressed by the time we were seated in Johan-

nesburg Airport waiting for someone to escort us to the plane. At last an unsmiling and bossy girl arrived. She pushed Peter's wheelchair so fast over the tarmac that I asked her to slow down, but she would not. The next minute the wheels hit a small pothole and Peter was flung out onto the ground. Several people came running, picked him up and back into the chair, shaken but basically unhurt. I was boiling with rage. I told the girl what her arrogant incompetence might have done, and I was not sorry I made her cry.

Once on the plane I hoped for a quiet flight home, but Peter drank two Martinis on a fairly empty stomach to "calm his nerves"; I couldn't deny that they might need calming, but unfortunately the meal was again long delayed. So it was sick-bag drill for the second time, and the situation did not remind me of those tempting advertisements to "fly the sunshine route to Africa" in which a happy couple are gaily toasting each other with the champagne served by a charming stewardess. However, we had enjoyed ourselves, Peter had almost a whole book under his belt, and the New Year 1978 was ahead with the hope of progress, always that hope of progress.

After the 1978 meeting of the Sloan-Kettering consultants, we took the opportunity to visit our youngest son, Alexander, in the Dutch West Indies. He was earning his living by acting as skipper, navigator, or electronic repair man on other people's boats while living on his own trimaran. He told us that life in the Caribbean was supposed to rot the soul; but his soul seemed to be all right. On our first day he borrowed a huge motor cruiser to take us to lunch on the French Island of St. Antoine. I was scared, wondering how the unwieldy boat could be managed if the big outboard motors broke down—there are no oars and no sail to fall back on. It was alarming getting Peter on board but all went well, and we were soon sitting out of doors in the sunshine at a small restaurant eating perfectly fresh fish, French bread and wine. The rest of the

few days went the same way and we flew home feeling good about
Alexander, especially because his teenage years had been so tire-
some.

In April, Peter and I decided that he could do without me for
ten days: I badly wanted to go to the Gambia, on the west coast of
Africa, to try out an audio-visual programme I had organised,
based on Barbara Ward's book *Only One Earth*. Barbara had been
invited by the United Nations to write a programme telling the
story of man's relations with his environment for people in developing countries. Because her health was fragile, she suggested I
should be invited instead, and I was delighted to accept. I thought
that the programme should first be tried out in a developing country, and when this was agreed I wrote a very simple text, based on
Barbara's book. Mark Boulton (of the International Centre for
Conservation Education) and I chose the pictures and I learnt all I
could about the Gambia from Mark, who had been there, and from
the people at the Gambian High Commission in London. We invited Alieu M'Boge from the High Commission to join us at home
for supper to help make plans for my visit. He told us that this was
the first time any member of the Gambian office had been entertained, as family, in an English home.

During the ten days I was away Peter went as usual every day
to his office, and when he came home was looked after by one or
other of the girls who had given us part-time help ever since his
first stroke in 1969. Every evening either a friend or one of the
family joined him for supper. By now we had a rota of three
helpers. Fiona was a very tall, blond speech therapist, Vicki was
a short, fair physiotherapist, and Elizabeth was a Guyanan occu-
pational therapist. Peter took them all to supper at Simpsons on
one of the evenings I was away. As the girls helped him up the
steps to the restaurant, the doorman said, "With respect, Sir, you
must have had a *very* interesting life. . . ."

He was right, except for the use of a past tense. In spite of his half vision, heavy splint and useless left arm, Peter was enjoying his work and life in general. He followed no special exercise routine—just climbing the stairs and hauling the heavy left leg around gave him plenty. He was now in much demand for lectures on his tumour-immunity work and almost as soon as I got home from the Gambia we started a round of visits to New York, Chicago, Brussels, Munich, St. Louis, and lastly Rome, for the International Transplant Conference.

The meetings were held in the Hilton Cavallieri Hotel, where we were comfortably installed in a big room with a balcony overlooking the city. On the first day of our stay, when we were sitting in the lobby before the next session of the conference began, a tall, balding man came up to us in a way I did not like—too deferential and too anxious to please. He introduced himself as an Italian transplant surgeon, practising in Rome. He told me, in a confidential voice, that he gave most of his money to support a hostel for nursing nuns in London, and that he frequently met and conversed with the Pope. After listening to more of such confidences, Peter switched off and began talking to someone else, but I was trapped. The surgeon asked me if I was aware of the different levels on which Life could be Lived. "You mean the physical, mental and moral?" I asked. He gasped. "Ah," he said, "then you *know,*" and gazed soulfully at both of us—then the next session of the conference saved me from more. Later on we learnt that this surgeon had been expecting to be elected as chairman of the European Chapter of the Society of International Transplant Surgeons. Instead, an English friend of ours had been chosen. That evening I met the friend on the stairs going into the dining room. He was upset and bewildered. "Do you know," he said, "I've just met Bellini [not his name] and he looked at me—and then cut me dead. What do you think this means?" Of course it meant that Bellini was furious because he had lost what he wanted. How unlike the English we thought, rather smugly.

Next day, all the members of the conference were invited to an audience with the Pope (John Paul I) in the audience hall of the Vatican. Peter scoffed a bit, expecting what he called "some sort of mumbo-jumbo." I said, "Just you wait." On this subject I knew him better than he knew himself.

We were not the only members of the public—the beautiful building, designed by Nervi, was almost full when our party was ushered into the front rows of hundreds and hundreds of chairs. Groups of nuns and pilgrims had come from all over Italy, each with an identifying banner. In front of us on a dais Vatican dignitaries in black were seated, keeping an eye on the choir boys in front of them. Finally the Pope entered and sat down on a high chair. A cleric read out the name of each group in the hall, and when the nuns had rustled to their feet, as moved and excited as schoolgirls, the Pope blessed them and spoke a few words. I felt they could hardly bear to sit down again; they would have liked their big moment, for which they had come so far, to have gone on for hours.

At last it was our turn, and a friend and I helped Peter to his feet for the blessing we were about to receive. Although it was in Italian, Peter's knowledge of opera librettos made it easy to understand, and I saw that his eyes were full of tears. I didn't whisper, "Some mumbo-jumbo."

When everybody had been blessed, the Pope came down from his dais and stopped beside our group. There was a small commotion at the end of the row in front of us, and I saw Bellini, on one knee, kissing the Pope's ring with great fervour while a photographer recorded his devotion. The result would certainly be hung on the wall of his surgery for the benefit of his patients.

Near the end of the ceremony, the Pope spoke to the choir boys. Then he called one to come forward. "And what is your name, my child?" The child replied clearly, "James"—not Giovanni, just James. The Pope asked him a few questions and then enquired how his mother was. James said she was in good health. The Pope became serious—what would James do if his mother should become ill? The expected answer was certainly that James should go down on his knees and pray to the Lord to make her well. But James was a practical child and he answered stoutly, "I and my brothers would look after her." The whole audience smiled, and so, to his credit, did the Pope, and James was allowed back to his seat without reproof.

It was a business to extricate ourselves, and Peter was tired from emotion and from sitting on the hard seat of the small chair. Mavi Marigonda, a friend of mine, was working in the Vatican for one of the bishops. I rang her office and with her help, the Vatican ambulance was called and made its way through the crowd to where we were waiting. We got Peter into it, and his arm sling was enough to indicate his status; but the driver and the attendant looked doubtfully at me. Then the driver said, "Lie down, signora, groan, and pretend you are to have a baby." In this way they drove us through the crowds, out of the big gate, and up the hill to the hotel where the porters greeted us, first with anxiety and then with shouts of delighted laughter.

Later on that week a treat was arranged for the delegates. We were to attend a concert in the Chapel of the Altar of Heaven—the Ara Coeli. The only way to reach the Ara Coeli was up a stone staircase of a hundred steps. Peter was keen to hear the music and as there were plenty of willing helpers around, I didn't veto the idea. We left plenty of time, took it easy, reached the top, got safely into the chapel and enjoyed the concert. Almost as the music ended there was a sound of steady drumming and then rushing water. I went to the door and looked out into a tropical rainstorm— the steps up to the Altar of Heaven had turned into a waterfall. Peter decided that he would rather descend in the rain than wait in the chapel where it had become quite cold. So we started. I stood behind him, holding his belt and guiding his uncertain left leg, a friend stood behind me, in case I slipped, a reporter appeared with an umbrella, and step by watery step we reached the bottom of the hundred stairs. There, Bellini was sitting in a car with his driver. He offered us a lift to the hotel; but he wanted to exclude the drenched friend who had helped us, on the grounds that he might make my dress wet. My hair was already as wet as if I had been swimming. I hauled the young man into the car as though I hadn't heard and wondered what the Pope would have thought of Bellini's charity.

The year 1979 was as busy as if Peter had no handicaps. He went to the Clinical Research Centre every day, planned research, reviewed books and wrote lectures; for variety there was an opera a month and a journey to Europe or America every other month. He was generous about my need for a break from responsibility and twice a year I had three or four days staying either in France with Caroline or Loulie or with a friend in the country. One of the girls who came in regularly to relieve me on one night a week would move in and take over, and I rang every evening to check that all was well.

At the end of July, Peter organised a small conference for immunologists and neurologists at the Villa Serbelloni. The weather was hot, humid and thundery, and one afternoon during one of the sessions Peter had a short and alarming period of amnesia; there were no apparent after-effects and the neurologists assured me that such attacks were often precipitated by these storms. For our summer holiday we had arranged to go on from Serbelloni to stay again at the Pflaums' hotel in Pegnitz for another *Ring* cycle at Bayreuth. I contacted a local doctor when we got there but there was really nothing he could do. He came all the same, examined Peter, and listened sympathetically but refused a fee; all he asked was an English pen-friend for his daughter.

Four months later we were invited to Riyadh in Saudi Arabia, where Peter was to lecture at the University Medical School. Riyadh must once have been an oasis, but now from the windows of the new luxury hotel in which we were staying the only trees I could see were single palm trees, their roots tied up in a ball, being unloaded into a row of holes beside the hotel entrance. Tall concrete buildings were everywhere growing up out of the dust. I kept my skirts long and my demeanour quiet, so the military doctor who was Peter's host allowed his wife, Sheik Yamani's sister, to come to a party and dinner with us.

She offered to show me the soukh market next day. I expected to find beautiful turquoise and silver ornaments and handwoven materials, but the stalls and their contents were mostly made in Birmingham. One of the doctors at the Medical School asked if there was anything I would like to do in Riyadh. I asked to see the unspoilt countryside outside the town and he drove us to the nearest point where there was water. The thin trickle in the sandy soil was just enough to nourish a bank of reeds; it was not like the oasis I had seen in picture books.

The plane returning us to London was delayed while the lavatories were unblocked. The last occupants, English and Americans working temporarily in Saudi Arabia, had drunk themselves unconscious on leaving Riyadh and had thoroughly blocked them. When we got home we found we had put on several pounds from drinking syrupy drinks instead of alcohol.

After eleven years without a stroke and with Peter's increasing strength and little loss of intellect, we felt less haunted in 1980— or anyway I did. I can't be sure what he felt. It was part of his nature not to waste time on fretting about something he couldn't influence. It was also just possible, as one neurologist had suggested, that there had been only one patch of weakness in the brain vessel which had ruptured from the high blood pressure in 1969. Since then I had regularly recorded the pressure and given very small doses of metaprolol if it rose—and this kept it at a pretty safe level. Our policy was to live as normally as we could without getting tired and not to refuse interesting invitations because of what might happen. The coward dies many deaths, the brave man dies but once.

TWELVE

Setback, 1980

THE NEXT BLOW FELL IN 1980 without warning. As we walked through the door into a party at the Clinical Research Centre, Peter hesitated and said, "I feel giddy." He sat down to drink a glass of water, but the giddiness persisted. We helped him to lie down on a couch in one of the hospital's examination rooms. Our friend Dr. Dom Pinto wanted him to stay the night, but this idea upset Peter—he insisted on going home, so after a while I drove him back, helped him go to bed and took his blood pressure. It was not high. He can't have felt well, though, because the next day he agreed not to go out to the Clinical Research Centre. Instead, he worked at home on the lecture he was to give eight days later at the Sloan-Kettering graduation ceremony in New York. That evening Solly Zuckerman came to dinner and there is a brief note in the diary, "Peter OK."

We had planned to go to New York via Paris for the wedding
party of Orly Abesirah, one of Peter's graduate research students.
Peter loved parties of colleagues, but after the giddy attack this
plan didn't seem sensible. He couldn't stand for long, party noise
confused him, and it was tiring to look up with only half his sight
at people who came to talk round his chair; so he reluctantly agreed
to cancel the Paris trip. Within a few days he seemed to have
recovered fully. The idea of cancelling the American trip and
letting down what was expected of him at the graduation ceremony
bothered him so much that it seemed safer, on balance, to take the
risk of possible consequences. We flew to New York and dined
that night at the Pierre Hotel with Otto Westphal, Lewis and Beryl
Thomas. It felt like old times and Peter responded with high spirits.

The graduation ceremony at Sloan-Kettering started at four
o'clock next day. I laid Peter's notes on the speaker's reading desk
so that he wouldn't have to carry them when he left his seat. He
began with exactly the right note for a formal but friendly occasion: quite a long quote from Sir Francis Bacon. Then he stopped
and said, with some surprise, that his notes were missing—perhaps they had been picked up by the previous speaker? This was
what had happened. The notes had lodged behind a paper clip, but
with apologetic laughter were soon retrieved and returned. The
applause for Peter's quoting from memory could not have been
greater had the situation been carefully stage-managed. Actually
the passage was one of those that moved him to tears so we had
gone over it many times until he felt less emotional.

The day after the ceremony the scientific consultants were to
meet all day. I asked one of them, Dr. Chester Stock, to keep an
eye on Peter and to arrange for him to have a break at midday.
Peter wouldn't agree. Chester said he contributed a lot to the
discussions.

In the evening Robert and Joanne Good gave a supper party in their penthouse on the sixteenth floor of the Sloan-Kettering building. We were in a very good mood as we arrived. Peter was happy because he knew he had made useful contributions to the discussions and had pleased everyone with the speech at the graduation ceremony. The view from the huge windows of the Goods' apartment was enough to put anyone in a relaxed mood. The skyscrapers blazed with points of light as if every window had a candle flickering behind the glass; inside the room, round tables were set out for dinner, drinks were being poured and everyone was welcoming Peter like a wounded hero.

He hardly responded as he sat sipping at a drink. After a few minutes he said, "I feel giddy again." As I looked at his face, I saw with alarm that his left eye was slewed towards his nose.

We helped him to lie down on Joanne's bed, where he stayed quietly for a few minutes; but soon he wanted to get up and go back to Abby Aldrich Hall. Bob Good organised a wheelchair from the hospital floor below us, we pushed Peter back over the road again and took the lift up to our room. I helped him to bed and he fell asleep. During the night his breathing sounded very thick, he had difficulty in swallowing, and by morning his speech was thick too. Various people at the party had assured me that the flu now going round made some people giddy, but as I listened to his breathing that night I knew that these stories had been just for comfort. I rang our old friend Dr. Jerry Lawrence early in the morning. He promised he'd be with us in about half an hour, would call an ambulance and ring Dr. Gerry Posner, the neurologist at Sloan-Kettering, to ask him to admit Peter into the intensive-care unit.

Jerry Lawrence arrived before the ambulance. When it came, the ambulance men thought this couldn't be the emergency they had expected, and if it was, they said, surely Sloan-Kettering

Memorial Cancer Hospital was not the place to go. "It is," Jerry said reverting to his naval officer voice, "and on my responsibility that is where we are going, fast."

I dreaded the idea of an intensive-care ward. Our ex-son-in-law, Loulie's husband, had once described the experience of being in one as "mind-blowing." But this ward wasn't mind-blowing at all. A pretty nurse welcomed us calmly and introduced herself as Ruth. She was the equivalent of an English Sister-in-Charge.

Very soon Peter was in bed on a saline and heparin drip. This time he had had a stroke in the brainstem, and his breathing, swallowing, and voice were affected. Dr. Posner took me into his office to hear Peter's history and invited me to use the room when I felt like it. He went off to telephone Michael Kremer in London while I looked at the pictures on the walls. One was of Kermit the Frog, his legs crossed one over the other, telephoning expansively to a colleague. "If you can't baffle them with science," he was saying, "blind them with bullshit." I laughed in spite of misery and went to tell the joke to Peter. He wanted to laugh too, only making the usual "ha-ha" wasn't possible; but I could see that the amusement did him good and I decided to collect more for him. When Dr. Chester Stock heard this on a visit to Peter he said, "You must have been reading *Anatomy of an Illness* by Norman Cousins." I hadn't, but when he gave me the book I was impressed. Norman Cousins's story that Vitamin C and laughter had arrested his normally fatal neurological disease is doubted or queried by some people; but if it had helped Norman Cousins and could do no harm, it might suit Peter. I was allowed to sleep in the hospital in a room used during the day by the consultants, so Peter had my constant familiar company as well as the excellent nursing.

The eleven years of slow climbing up from the effects of the first stroke had been long enough to induce a feeling of some security. Now the new shock was both numbing and terrifying. My heart beat so hard and so fast in the first twenty-four hours that

I was exhausted and slept without moving in the uncomfortable bed. Dorothy Lawrence came daily from 30th to 67th Street with a supply of fresh orange juice. Peter called it "ambrosia." Her kindness was a tonic for me and very good for Peter.

Family and friends are essential in crises. We were surrounded by them, both new and long standing ones. Charles and his wife Caroline were in America and came to New York, and Alexander flew up from his sailing business in St. Maarten. They were both quietly and steadily helpful, and I enjoyed more time with them than we could have had in London. Herman Wouk rang regularly and David Pyke re-routed one of his lecture assignments in America to come to the hospital, see Peter, and bolster my morale. The Goods lent me a room in their apartment so I could be rung from London in privacy.

On the first night Peter was in hospital, Dr. Laird Myers, the Dean of the hospital and till then a stranger, invited me home for supper to meet his family. It was very comforting to be welcomed into normal family life; this one included a new grandchild to admire, analgesic alcohol and a very good dinner. During the five weeks Peter was in hospital in New York I was never alone for an evening meal. American hospitality and kindness is unbeatable.

After ten days in the intensive-care unit, Dr. Posner was surprised and delighted by Peter's improvement: he began to breathe and swallow more normally, smiled crookedly and croaked remarks. At first I had been told "anything" could happen. I couldn't and dared not believe this. I fed him into the right side of his mouth, with no more than half a teaspoon of orange juice or he choked. As his swallowing improved, he began moving the left leg and exercising his hand with five-finger exercises. He was often extremely tired, so tired that his voice was not much more than a loud whisper, but he could still joke and enjoy other people's humour. He actually laughed out loud when Dr. Posner told him that Teilhard de Chardin, who had died recently, had "gone to study higher consciousness above."

After two weeks he was moved from intensive care into Room 728, and a cot for me was added. I wondered if this concession would upset the nursing staff. Jerry Posner said it wouldn't be-cause we were a tonic for them— Peter was getting better and most of the acute cancer patients weren't. The room was not really made for two beds; Peter called it a "high-class oubliette."

At first, being responsible for Peter at night kept me awake. It wasn't safe to leave him for long in the day, because he couldn't turn in bed and he found using the call bell very difficult—his voice wasn't strong enough to be effective through the wall micro-phone. Once, he did use it, and when I asked what he had said, he replied, "I called out 'Wolf, wolf' as loudly as I could," and choked with laughter.

Towards the end of two months, when Dr. Lewis Thomas came to visit Peter, he mentioned that if our medical insurance did not cover the hospital bills, we were not to worry. "You are one of us, Peter," he said. But, for fear of trouble, I had insured both with the Medical Research Council and privately, so we were all right, and so was the hospital.

Peter was knocked out by this stroke, and besides losing most of his voice, he had to learn to walk all over again. He began to try to put one foot in front of the other in the basement gym, helped by the hospital's physiotherapist, Eileen Bach. She was good to look at, even from the close quarters required by physiotherapy, intelligent and understanding—so Peter's progress between par-allel bars was not the usual gymnastic penance. By the end of April he was thought well enough to travel and walk a few steps, using his stick. We hired an ambulance to take us to the airport. Two strong young men arrived on time, settled Peter in a comfort-able front seat, and welcomed the party who were seeing us off: Dorothy, Jean Nimkin (the best and kindest fixer I have ever met) and Alexander. Halfway to Kennedy one of the ambulance men asked kindly, "Like some milk, Pete?" When we reached the aircraft they lifted Peter bodily into his seat on the British Airways plane; then they cheerfully kissed me goodbye as if they were affectionate relatives.

We slept through the overnight journey, thanks to a small sleeping pill and the promise of the steward to wake me if Peter needed my help as well as his. In the early morning at Heathrow another ambulance crew met us, briefed to drive us to a side ward for two at Northwick Park Hospital. There we spent another eight weeks of sheltered life under the kind care of Dr. Robert Mahler. The ward was only a corridor away from Peter's small team in the Clinical Research Centre; one of the team, the German neurologist Jürgen Mertin, came in early every morning to help me get Peter up and dressed and exercised. Later, the other members, Liz Simpson, Ruth Hunt and Joy Heys, visited him in turn and kept him up to date on the progress of experiments and with letters that had to be answered.

One of the letters contained an invitation from Ronny Schwartz. Ever since Bernard Schwartz's death, Ronny had been planning ways of celebrating his life. She arranged exhibitions of the Outstanding Features portraits in the Kennedy Center and all over America. Perhaps the best known of the portraits is the one of Lord Mountbatten in full naval uniform and full profile—a profile that was, as I heard one woman say gazing up at it, "enough to knock your socks off." Ronny's letter told us that she had decided to found a memorial lecture, at the University Medical School at La Jolla in California, and she invited Peter to deliver it in the autumn of 1980. Ronny's invitation came with every inducement to accept, though in spite of the distance to be travelled we did not need inducements. Peter was improving and he still had three months in which to build up strength—and he was elated and challenged to be asked.

Ronny made comfortable travel arrangements for October, and

we flew the long haul to Los Angeles without anxiety. A car of generous size met us and soon we were settled in the Schwartz guest house in San Diego, within sound of the Pacific Ocean. Ronny had thought of everything; the huge refrigerator was stocked with fresh orange juice, fruit, vegetables, chicken and cheeses, enough for a week. We spent nine extremely pleasant days with her. Apart from Peter's lecture he had no duties, and the visit became a holiday. She gave a party for us at her house on cliffs overlooking a rocky cove; she provided a chess player and even a medical student to be with Peter while Jonas Salk took me either for a walk or a swim in the ocean. He gave a party at his house and showed us all over his Institute, the most beautiful modern building I have ever seen. This visit made Peter regret a little that he had once turned down an invitation to work there for a while. At the time he had felt the "while" to be too long and the situation perhaps too isolated.

In addition to everything else, Ronny invited Gwyneth Jones to fly down from San Francisco where she was singing *Turandot* at the opera house. It was a beautiful and well-staged surprise. Gwyneth took this opportunity to suggest that Peter should go to a healer called Olga Stringfellow. This healer, she said, had almost instantly repaired the damage to her arm which the wicked operatic character Hunding had caused when he gripped her too fiercely while throwing her to the ground in an exaggerated jealous fury. Gwyneth is a girl of imagination and faith. I am more sceptical, but about the healing effect of Gwyneth on Peter I was not sceptical. I told her how shallow Peter's breathing was, and how he needed to improve it for his lecture. Would she consider giving him a lesson in using his diaphragm, lungs and voice in unison? Of course she would. "Put your hand here, Peter," she said, guiding his willing hand to her diaphragm and then, as Peter said afterwards, "she began to swell alarmingly." I don't know how the rest of the lesson went, because I went off to swim, but the whole treatment probably rivalled anything Miss Stringfellow might have accomplished.

While we were away, I had arranged for our builder, Mr. Price, to alter the house so that Peter need not climb to the top floor for bed. Mr. Price and three Jamaican friends were to make a bedroom and bathroom on the first floor, where our sitting room and study had been, and to turn the ground-floor passage and bed sitting room on the floor below into a kitchen and dining room. This could be done only by cutting a large oblong shape in the wall which was common to the passage and future dining room. Anyone who has lived through construction work will remember that no matter how many dust sheets and how many newspapers are used, the fine plaster dust can penetrate even a screwtop lid and into a honey pot. Furthermore, two radiators had to be moved and reconnected in different places.

We arrived home at last and opened the front door, longing to be back in our altered house and to congratulate Mr. Price on what he had accomplished. All we could see was dust and all we could feel was cold. Mr. Price emerged, from the dust cloud, white with plaster and looking miserable. He had worked until eleven o'clock the night before, trying to trace a lost connection under the floorboards—without it he couldn't put on the heating. The situation was so awful we could only laugh and commiserate with him. Mrs. Brown had managed to clean one room and the beds had been moved into it. So we turned on the electric fan heaters, warmed it up, ate a picnic and fell asleep.

In the next days Mr. Price and his mates worked overtime. When they finished the job, the house fitted us again and the bill was a fraction of what it would have cost to move.

Nothing that happened in 1981 gave more pride and joy than a document informing Peter that the Queen had awarded him the Order of Merit—the highest of all civil orders. Of course someone draws the Queen's attention, if need be, to a man or woman who might fittingly join the Order, limited to twenty-four, when a place becomes available through a death. An inscribed parchment duly arrived, in which Her Majesty referred to Peter as her "trusty and well beloved servant," and we were invited to Buckingham Palace for the investiture, on 27 February, our forty-fourth wedding anniversary. The arrangements made by the Palace included the posting of a strong equerry at the foot of the steps leading into the hall, ready to give help if needed. We were ushered into a large ante chamber, overlooking the gardens; if you didn't know you were in the middle of London, you could imagine you were looking out at a well-established garden in the heart of Surrey. Two other men had been chosen to join the Order: Lord Olivier and Sir Leonard Cheshire, the heroic wartime pilot and founder of the Cheshire homes for the disabled. Leonard Cheshire had been "done" the day before and Laurence Olivier's turn was after Peter's—M comes before O. While we waited we talked to him about a mutual friend, the publisher Hamish Hamilton, at whose ball Laurence Olivier had danced with me, years before. "Couldn't do it now," he said ruefully.

Presently the door to the Queen's drawing room opened and we saw her standing beside three chairs and a small table, on which was lying the box holding the Order of Merit. The Queen does her job perfectly. She is clearly in gentle and charming command, and if you weren't loyal subjects before meeting her, as we were, you would become one.

Later, the Queen gave a lunch for the members of the Order and their wives at Windsor Castle. Just before 10:00 p.m. the night before the lunch the telephone rang. Sir Philip Moore, the Queen's private secretary, apologised for ringing late but Her Majesty had wondered if I should sit on Sir Peter's left at the lunch or whether it would be in order to seat a member of the household beside him. We admired the Queen's thoughtfulness. I replied that I need not sit on his left but that I would be grateful if whoever they chose instead might be briefed about the handicaps and to keep an eye on Peter's needs at table.

We had never been to Windsor Castle. Outside and inside it is just what a royal castle should be—imposing, impregnable, full of ancient history and modern comfort. As we walked slowly towards the room in which the Queen and Prince Philip were receiving their guests, I longed to stop and look at the paintings on the walls and at the glass cases of china and books. Peter and ex-Prime Minister Sir Harold Macmillan were both walking with a stick and Sir Harold was going slightly faster; Peter's sister Pamela had met Sir Harold when her first husband, Sir David Hunt, was the Prime Minister's secretary, so the families were slightly acquainted.

As he caught up with us, Sir Harold straightened up slightly, surveyed the scene and commented, "Proper old people's outing I call it, my dear."

The lunch was held in the Waterloo Room, hung with oil portraits of the generals who had fought on the 1815 battlefield. Somebody told me that when General de Gaulle had been entertained in the Waterloo Room, named after the battle in which his countryman Napoleon had been defeated, the General made a very dry French remark. I remember laughing and thinking that I would never forget the story, but I did and had to chase it up. On being shown the many portraits of the English generals, de Gaulle commented, *"Tiens, il fallait tous ces gens là pour battre Napoléon!"* (Imagine, so many generals needed to fight Napoleon!)

I sat between Sir Kenneth Clark and Sir Frederick Ashton and much enjoyed their company. Luckily I had just read Sir Kenneth's book *Civilisation* for the third time, so I could appear better informed than I would have been had we met the month before. Sir Frederick the choreographer seemed pleased that I thought ballet ranked as an art form. "Most people," he said, "think, an Order of Merit for service to the ballet—how inappropriate!"

At odd times during 1981 I noticed that Peter was either seeing worse or becoming absent-minded. One evening, as we came home from the opera, I parked the car in Downshire Hill, a few doors away from our house in the terrace. While I locked the car, Peter walked slowly on, straight past our house, which he should have recognised because the front railings were the only ones covered with roses. I suggested a visit to the oculist for stronger glasses but he didn't take to the idea and we put it off. Then in November the Royal College of Physicians arranged a symposium on Disabilities, to be conducted by three people who had them, Peter being one. Lady Masham described how she managed her life from a wheelchair, and Dr. Charles Fletcher recounted some of his experiences as a diabetic. "Darling, I think I'm going," he had desperately called to his wife as his blood sugar dropped to an alarming level. "Yes, darling," she had calmly replied, "but first wait a minute and take your glucose"—after which he returned from the feeling of imminent dissolution to normal life.

In his contribution, Peter briefly described the seventeen years since his first stroke at age fifty-three. He said that his decided preference for staying alive was the strongest force pulling him back to a normal life. As usual he made a light and amusing story out of daunting handicaps and setbacks. At the dinner afterwards, instead of sitting beside him as I usually did, I was placed opposite where I had a close view of his left eye. I felt a pang of alarm— something was really wrong with it. It looked red and sore and was bulging slightly. After the dinner I asked David to recommend an eye specialist who would see Peter at once. Shortly after we got home, Mr. David Abrams arrived. He examined Peter's eyes very carefully and then said gently, "You don't see very well out of this eye, do you?"

Peter agreed and I guessed that what Mr. Abrams was saying was that the left eye was blind. We made an appointment to see him in the local hospital and there, two days later, his diagnosis was confirmed. The eye was suffering from glaucoma—increased internal pressure. We were given drops and made an appointment to come back in a few weeks time. Luckily Peter did not have the headaches many people suffer with this condition.

His sight was now down to one half of the right eye. I bought a very bright light and with this he was able to read, though not for long. His vision was already so restricted that he hadn't noticed the extra loss. There aren't many compensations for such loss, but it was lucky that most of Peter's pleasures came from imagining and thinking. He enjoyed beauty, but not for long at a time. For example, he found constant urging to appreciate the fall colours by kind American hosts in autumn visits a bit trying. "Once you've seen one set of Fall Colours," he said (to me, not to them), "you've seen them all."

Before his stroke slowed him down, Peter had never been keen on weekend visits to friends' houses. He liked being at home and having time to read, play chess against an automatic player Alexander had given him or listen to the gramophone or tapes. He made an exception once or twice and we stayed with Victor and Tess Rothschild in Cambridge in the quiet luxury which money alone cannot buy. Victor's butler, Sweeny, was an especial attraction because he remembered exactly what every guest liked to drink before dinner, and how much. Victor said that he valued Sweeny (who had been his batman during the war) far more than he did his children, and Tess threatened that if Sweeny ever left, she would leave too.

On one of our visits, Lady Diana Cooper was also staying. Victor asked her what period of her life she had most enjoyed. "When I acted the Nun in Reinhardt's production of *The Miracle*," she replied. Victor gave a mock groan. "God," he said, "I was afraid so." Lady Diana preserved her remarkable beauty by staying late in bed in the morning with her lap dog, called Doggie. She thought Peter was very beautiful, as he was, and told him so— which of course he didn't mind. At lunch one day a bottle of claret was circulated. Peter and I tasted it, marvelled, and looked at one another. Then Peter asked the vintage. "Oh that," said Victor, "it's what we call *un petit vin de famille.*"

Peter was now much more sociable than he had been before his stroke—he had more time. We were invited to stay at Eyeford House in the Cotswolds where Sir Cyril and Lady Kleinwort had arranged the sort of hospitality that reminded me of descriptions of Edwardian country house parties. The greyish-gold Cotswold stone house is set in rolling parkland planted with huge trees. The River Eye runs through the grounds and forms two dark lakes. A pair of geese return every year to nest on an island in the middle, in spite of persecution by resident foxes. The garden, largely designed by Betty Kleinwort, is the sort that keen gardeners visit with notebooks and cries of delight.

Meals were cooked and served by a talented young woman and the wines were chosen by Betty's son-in-law. In the evenings she arranged bridge games for Peter's entertainment. He hadn't played since Mama died, and now had only one functioning hand and less than half his eyesight. We propped his cards in a holder designed by the Therapy Department at Northwick Park Hospital; to my delight, and his, he managed not to let his partner down and everyone was happy.

At Eyeford Betty arranged that Peter could dictate in peace in a small drawing room, overlooking the terrace to the hills beyond. There was a wood fire, bowls of flowers, paintings by Boldini and Augustus John and shelf after shelf of books. In these surroundings he finished dictating a new book called *The Limits of Science.** Its theme stressed that science should not be expected to provide solutions to problems such as the purpose of life or the existence of God, for which it was unfitted.

On a later visit Betty showed me a thank-you letter from a

*(New York: Harper & Row, 1984).

young woman who had been one of the bridge players. In a P.S. she had added that Peter was the bravest and most remarkable man she had ever met.

Shortly after this Eyeford visit we left for Boston, where Harvard University was to award Peter an honorary degree. The honour gave him a lot of pleasure; he also had the minor pleasure of collecting an H for Harvard for his game of Alphabetical Academic Awards. When he listed them in *Memoir of a Thinking Radish,* he noted that Yale was, "like Zimbabwe, alas, unaccountably dragging its feet" in not providing a Y and a Z respectively.

Among the other honorary graduates were Mother Teresa and Tennessee Williams. At the end of a splendid ceremony arranged under a marquee in the Harvard Yard, I noticed that a burly figure approached Mother Teresa and gently bundled her off the platform, before the rest of the party broke up. When I asked the meaning of this kidnap, I was told that at a similar ceremony the poor lady had had her garments rent by people eager to have a piece of the cloth from the habit she was wearing.

At the party afterwards I saw Mother Teresa sitting on a bench beside her attendant nun. She looked a little lonely, so I went to speak to her. She promptly blessed me, as she did anyone who came near her. I thought it might interest her to bless Peter—she would not have known his views on some aspects of her religion—so I showed her where he was sitting in his wheelchair. She kindly officiated and he enjoyed her kindness; but he was also longing for a drink. So when Tennessee Williams appeared, he explained that Mother Teresa had just blessed him and added, "Now, Mr. Williams, what are you going to do for me?" Mr. Williams knew at once. "I'll get you a drink," he said, and hurried through the crowd to collect one from the bar.

When we got home in May, the proofs of Peter's new book *From Aristotle to Zoos* arrived. This was the light-hearted encyclopaedia of biological terms, chosen mainly because they amused or interested him. The one I liked best was his description of a virus: "A piece of bad news, wrapped in protein." As he watched Peter dictating entries, David Pyke once asked him how much more he still had to do; Peter grinned and said simply, "I'll know when I've finished." He dictated into his small hand-held machine, straight out of his head, and only occasionally asked me to verify a point. Joy Heys typed the tapes and then he and I went through the pages. Sometimes I shut my left eye and covered half of my right as I read, to remind myself what reading was like for Peter. The handicap was exceedingly frustrating, but he grumbled only occasionally, claiming that the light was bad. Apart from the eye he looked very well and we managed the usual programme of laboratory work, travel, operas, writing and meals with and for friends. He enjoyed what he called his "vittles," and I worried about his weight in case it strained his heart. We went several times for checkups to Sir Richard Bayliss. Richard checked that all systems were in order and then stared like a headmaster at Peter. "You will lose at least a stone, Peter," he said, and this had an effect for a while, during which 7 lbs were slowly lost.

The eye unfortunately wasn't responsive to the eyedrops prescribed for glaucoma, and by January 1984 Mr. Abrams was worried by its condition—the cornea was in a bad state and likely to become infected. In his opinion Peter would do well to be rid of it. There is something sickening about the idea of having an eye removed, and both Dick Bayliss and Mr. Abrams warned that many people became very upset at the idea. Peter was bravely practical; the eye was no asset, the operation was supposed to be quick and simple, so "let's get on with it" was his reaction.

We booked into a side ward of the Royal Free Hospital in Hampstead at the beginning of February and I moved in as an extra nurse. I brought with me the seventeen-year record of Peter's blood pressure so that the anaesthetist could judge what medication would be appropriate before and during the operation.

Instead of twenty to thirty minutes, Peter was in the operating theatre for two and a half hours. Waiting in these circumstances is intolerable—you don't know what is wrong and there is nobody to ask because they are all in the theatre. At last Mr. Abrams came out: he looked both grim and relieved. He explained that Peter's blood pressure had soared under the anaesthetic and until the resultant haemorrhage was controlled the operation could not start.

Peter was terribly restless in the night that followed. I stayed until late, but Loulie stayed all night, on a makeshift bed of chairs, saying, "He'll need you tomorrow," and it was good that she did, because he was very confused. He kept on wanting to get rid of the bandages over his eye. In the morning when I arrived, the anaesthetist met me in the corridor. "Next time he has to have an operation," she said blandly, "it would be a good idea to have an anti-hypertensive dose before." Luckily for her, my governess-trained temper prevented me from seizing her and shaking the idea into her head that it was her responsibility, not mine, to assess what medication the patient should have—and that I had brought the blood pressure charts precisely in order to help her to decide. The long anaesthesia, during which the brain is actually poisoned into insensibility, did Peter no good at all.

After four days we left the Royal Free and went out to Northwick Park Hospital, where we shared a room on Galen Ward, again thanks to our friend Dr. Robert Mahler, the physician in charge. In this way Peter kept in touch with his work in the Clinical Research Centre, separated only by one floor and several corridors. Ruth Hunt continued with the experiments they had designed and Peter looked forward to her visits and progress reports.

In March he acquired a lifelike eye—"beer-bottle brown," his mother would have called it, and his directions to the eye maker recalled her description—"beer-bottle brown, with a merry twinkle, please." Thanks to cunning arrangements by Mr. Abrams, the eye could be moved from side to side and it fooled most people.

When I put it back after washing it, Peter often claimed he could see better, and this joke anyway amused us.

We had a quick visit to Toronto towards the end of the month and went on to Chapel Hill and the Grahams; the excuse for staying again with the Grahams was an invitation to me from Dr. Malcolm Potts's Family Health International organisation, to show an audio-visual presentation I had arranged on the relation between people and the environment. The technician had telephoned me in London to check that their machine fitted my video cassette, but as the audience was getting comfortably settled he appeared with a gloomy face, to tell me that my video and his machine did not after all match together. All I could do was to remember the text and ask the audience to close their eyes and imagine the pictures I was describing. They were very good at this and somehow the evening did not seem wasted. Peter claimed to have enjoyed it.

During the next few days in Chapel Hill he began feeling unwell and developed a low fever. John Graham summoned their family physician, Dr. Bill Yount. He was ideal—calm but concerned. He began, endearingly, by asking Peter *his* views on the diagnosis, which made them both laugh. Whatever the cause was, the symptoms passed off and we flew home and spent Easter peacefully with Betty Kleinwort at Eyeford.

In July the Mahlers invited us to Glyndebourne to hear the opera *Così fan tutte*. Bill Hoffenberg, the President of the Royal College of Physicians, and his wife completed the party. It was the sort of evening that advertisers set up in order to persuade you to buy whatever they want to sell. The opera was enchanting, the gardens were at their best, and the air smelt of lilies, freshly cut grass and woodsmoke. I had packed a good picnic, based on cold roast guinea fowl, and the Hoffenbergs kept up a stream of champagne. Normally I should have been absorbed by happiness, but although Peter was able to walk with the aid of his stick he couldn't manage to get up from his seat in the interval. We hoisted him up under each arm; but I remember hoping this was a stage in his recovery and not a downward trend.

Our last foreign trip was to Seattle. I went ahead for a few days' holiday and Peter bravely followed, boarding and disembarking by accompanied wheelchair. We met at Kennedy Airport and stayed the night in New York before crossing to the West Coast. In Seattle, he gave his last lecture. There was a very appreciative audience and we were most kindly entertained. Arno and Gretel Motulsky gave us a welcoming lunch in their home. I remember that the food was delicious, but not what it was, because what made the lunch particularly memorable was Peter's eye falling out with a clatter onto his plate. I murmured something about it being a good thing to be among friends when performing that old trick and Peter behaved with unselfconscious grace, as he always did whenever something physically embarrassing occurred.

He had planned the last lap of the journey as a treat. We were to stay in the Westbury Hotel in New York and sail home on the *Queen Elizabeth 2*. For the first time, I found I couldn't safely manage helping Peter by myself. There were too many near-misses as we transferred from standing to a chair or bed. So instead of the gala supper he had planned in the hotel restaurant downstairs, we had a quiet meal in our room. I rang the Lawrences for help. Of course they immediately invited us to stay in their apartment and by evening we had transferred and I felt much safer. Next day I learnt that the *QE2* had no wheelchair. Dorothy helped me to hire one (Peter protested but I knew we needed it). The Lawrences came to see us off, a band played lively music, a photographer took jolly photographs and we found we had a comfortable cabin and bathroom, sizes larger than the one on the banana boat in 1970. Although our cabin was near the lifts, the passages were too long for Peter to walk without getting very tired, so we covered most of the distances by wheelchair. I pushed him as far as the door of the restaurant, he managed to walk from it to our table, and the waiters folded up the wheelchair out of the way.

The advertisements for the *QE2* are full of gastronomic clichés—the genre of "fresh butter from the mountains," "tender morsels of fillet steak robed in Béarnaise sauce," "crisp salads," and so on. Considering the amount of food that has to be frozen and can't be served fresh from the farm, the meals were creditable, but gourmet, no. Peter said the style was exactly as if one of the large Atlantic City hotels had been pushed out to sea. The company was not what it used to be or is supposed to be. The party at the table next to ours, and very much within earshot, found life on the *QE2* suited them perfectly. I heard their life story: the principal lady was the widow of a provincial newspaper proprietor who had left her well off and this, she told us, was her nineteenth cruise. There was bridge and Bingo and hairdressing, shops and television and gambling, so she found never a dull moment; but after the introductory recitation, her conversation was limited.

On the second day in the late afternoon all the lights went out and the hum of the engines stopped. We were in the cabin and it wasn't yet quite dark. The captain's voice came over the intercom. There had been some trouble in the engine room, he explained—we later learnt that an explosion had burnt one of the crew and put him into sick bay—but this was being attended to, and we would in due course be on our way again. In the meantime he begged everyone to remain calm and to avoid going to one side of the ship all at the same time. The idea of what might happen if we all did was unpleasantly emphasised by the increasing slow roll of the ship. It was best not to look out of the porthole at the level of the horizon, slowly disappearing and reappearing as the ship righted herself. After a while it grew dark. I made my way to the dining room where stewards had put shaded candles on each table. It wasn't our dining room so I didn't know the steward, but I asked him if I might borrow a light, because the thought of Peter trying to get into the bathroom in the dark alarmed me. The steward said no, he couldn't spare one, so I waited until he had gone and then made off with it.

At regular intervals the captain's voice returned, and as each time he said exactly the same thing, it was not reassuring. I had got so fed up with our table neighbours that I consulted the passenger list for possible company. To my joy I found General Sir John Hackett's name, accompanied by his family. Meeting them changed everything for the better. Sir John diagnosed exactly what had happened when the accident was reported to the captain. "When they gave him the news," he said, "the captain fell on the deck in a dead faint. They wrote out this bulletin, two jolly Jack Tars propped him upright, and he's been reading it out at regular intervals ever since."

The bulletins stopped the next morning and we arrived in Southampton only a day late. Our friend, the author Peter Gibson, was waiting at the dock to drive us back in his car to Hampstead.

THIRTEEN

Losing Ground, 1984

 S THE DECADES PASS, the perspective on death short-
ens. The earlier "Oh well, needn't think about that
just yet" shifts to "I I'm, three score and ten, perhaps
I'd better start thinking."

Our American friends, Dorothy and Jerry Lawrence, began
thinking in plenty of time. They chose a plot in a small country
churchyard in Connecticut for their grave. Dorothy instructed her
children to remember that she hoped to find a large bottle of her
favourite dinner-time drink, "hearty red burgundy," inside her
coffin, to refresh her on her way to the shades. Every time they
passed this last resting place, she expressed her appreciation; she
did this so often that Jerry finally stopped the car and suggested
that, as she found it so attractive, they might like to stop and take
up residence ahead of time.

Their forethought decided me to follow their example. I don't like cremation; I prefer that the elements from which we are made should be recycled instead of transformed by a burst of electricity into polluting smoke.

When I told Peter of the Lawrences' plan, his eyes filled with tears. When you love, you have a "hostage to fortune" and the idea of separation is not tolerable. I tried to cheer us up, not very successfully. Peter suddenly came up with a typical solution. "I know," he said. "Don't let's . . ." and then we couldn't help laughing. He had his preference for remaining alive and I did all I could to make it worthwhile. He told a friend, visiting at this time, "She rejoices in keeping me alive."

All was going comparatively well until the morning of Sunday 9 June 1985. When Peter woke, he asked me in a weak voice what day it was. I told him, but he forgot the answer within a minute and kept on asking again. Something was badly wrong. I hoped the trouble might be a transient attack of global amnesia, which he had had before. It wasn't. Our friend Dr. John Newsom Davis came that afternoon. He decided that, if Peter wasn't better by the evening, he would admit him the next day to the National Hospital in Queen Square. By Monday Peter wasn't better, and we called the ambulance. As we drove I put my arm round him and each time he asked where we were going, I said that it was for a check visit to the hospital. He would seem to understand for a few minutes, and then his face would again crumple, puzzled about what was happening.

The brain scan showed more damage in the brainstem from another stroke. Peter was so ill that John told David Pyke that he thought Peter had begun his last illness. He told Loulie that the amount of damage was so large that it was impossible to understand how Peter had been managing any sort of life at all, let alone writing his memoir and working in the Clinical Research Centre every weekday.

I don't know how to describe the cold, sick misery of this time. It coloured everything with a grey haze. You go through a day in which there is no normal routine—everything hangs on what is happening to Peter in that hospital bed. Early training, by sensible precepts, helped a little: don't give up hope, go to bed early, keep warm, don't drink too much tea and take some time away from the hospital; all boring advice, but I took it.

Peter was nursed in a corner bed of the big ward, just beside the Sister's room. He was on a drip and was only semi-conscious. I held his hand a lot of the time and slept in a small spare room on the top floor of the hospital. Caroline and Charles and Loulie came in relays to be with him, and when I went to bed at night Loulie stayed up beside him until 3:00 a.m. Then I came down and she went upstairs to sleep in the still-warm bed.

Against all fears Peter very gradually improved—but he couldn't see. Sometimes he murmured out loud and Caroline made notes of what he said. Once, Loulie heard him whisper, *"Requiescat in pace"*—but he wasn't ready to give up his very decided preference, and within a few days the physiotherapist began working with him. Soon they managed to transfer him to a wheelchair and into the gym. There I saw him one morning, sitting on the edge of a treatment couch, supported from behind by the physiotherapist who was encircling him with her arms and encouraging him to breathe deeply. I stood in front of him without speaking and after a moment he lifted his head, smiled faintly, and said, "I've had another stroke, haven't I?" What could I say? I said yes—but that he was making extraordinary progress and he smiled again, more strongly.

The progress was slow and erratic, but it was progress, and after a month we found that he still had some tunnel vision in the remaining eye. Loulie's daughter, Siiri, noticed that when she put a dark cherry on a white tissue on his supper tray, Peter pounced on it and ate it. She moved it into different positions on the white background, testing how much he could see. This discovery brought tremendous relief: from then on we played at reading games, taken from the large-print notices on the wall of the ward or on cornflake packets. As long as Peter remembered that his eye would read "CORNFLAKES" as "ORNFLAKES" he did quite well. We began to practise with the newspaper headlines. It tired him after a few minutes, but it gave him hope.

One afternoon he said to me, "You know, people look at you with a new respect when you have been *there* and back." I knew he was referring to the River Styx, over which the boatman Death ferries people to the other world, so I asked, "Did you meet that old bugger with the scythe?" Peter laughed out loud. "Yes." "Well, what did you say?" He thought a moment and then said, pointing a valedictory finger, "I said, 'Avaunt!' " I wanted more. "Well, what was he doing?" Again the slight pause, and then he laughed— "He was picking his teeth with his scythe."

Visitors began to come to see him and help him with meals and stories, to encourage him or tell him jokes. The physiotherapists helped him with endless patience and he began to take a few steps. To their alarm, he and I took to climbing up the stairs—he holding hard on the bannisters and leaning his weight on them, almost over the stairwell below. We never tried it unless a friend stood behind me, as I steadied Peter firmly by his belt, but it looked alarming. Nevertheless, the achievement of accomplishing first two steps and then more each day until he reached the landing gave his morale the progress he craved in whatever he did.

By the spring of 1986 it was possible to consider what sort of a future we could plan. Sister Hill had convinced me at one point that it would not be possible for me to look after Peter at home, even though I was partially looking after him in hospital. He did some physio in the morning, had lunch and a long siesta. When I came in around 5:00 p.m. we went by wheelchair into the garden of Queen Square, or we tried reading large-print books. I helped him with supper and walking, undressing and getting into bed. Loulie came after he was in bed around nine most evenings and read to him. Family and friends visited regularly and helpfully.

I started finding out about stair lifts, bath hoists, district nursing and private nursing. I got a list of nursing homes, in case there was one near, with a resident physiotherapist, which Peter might use for three or four days a week and could then spend long weekends at home. None of them fitted and the stair lift didn't either. A conference was arranged at the hospital consisting of Dr. Michael Modell (our doctor), the hospital social workers and district nurses, and Sister Hill, to work out what could be managed in the way of help at home. The district nurses were charming and helpful, but of course they couldn't promise to come at any special time, and we wanted to start the day at a regular time with all the bathing business out of the way.

In the end by the sort of chance that happens if you exhaust everyone you meet with enquiries, David Duncan, an ex-army male nurse, highly recommended, came to see us at the hospital. We arranged with him that he would arrive at our house at about eight at night and stay the night, then in the morning he would help Peter to get washed and dressed and into a reclining chair for the day.

The problem now was how Peter could move about in a house arranged on four floors. He was still unsteady and could walk only a step or two. Until he could manage the stairs he would have to live in the second-floor bedroom and bathroom, away from the books and music in the floor below, and from the kitchen and dining room on the floor below that.

The generosity of the Kleinwort family solved the problem. I had worked with the head of the family, Sir Cyril Kleinwort, in raising money for the Family Planning International Campaign and during this time he developed a great admiration for Peter. Remembering this, his family decided to give us the magnificent present of a lift that would run up through the house, from the dining room, past the sitting room and up into the bedroom. Without this gift and David Duncan's tireless help, living at home would not have been possible.

By August 1986 the dirt raised by installing the lift through two floors had been patiently swept up and dusted off by Mrs. Brown. After a year and two months we said goodbye to Queen Square and the staff who had helped Peter back to life. By now I understood why this hospital was a Mecca for neurologists from all over the world. The buildings weren't new but the best of modern medicine was practised within them, and encouragement was always an important part of the way it was practised.

Although Peter's sight was limited to tunnel vision in the right eye, he could walk a few steps; together he and I could manage the transfer from bed to wheelchair, into the lift, and then from wheelchair into the car, so we would be able to go out for entertainment.

After we had settled down to the new routine at home we went every Saturday to Trattoria San Giorgio, a small Italian restaurant in Hampstead run by Franco and two helpers. There we had home-cooked food and a warm welcome. Even if it was snowing Franco put on his coat, left his customers, and came out to help us come in with the wheelchair, assuring us convincingly that it was a pleasure.

By November I felt it was safe to accept an invitation to Montreux from Professor Otto Westphal, to celebrate his remarriage* and to meet again his four-year-old son Alexander, my German godson. Otto Westphal was a great admirer of Peter's and we had stayed several times with him in Freiburg when he was head of the Max Planck Institute. Peter had enormously enjoyed giving informal lectures to students and especially to listening to accounts of their work afterwards. He was always a popular lecturer in Europe

---

* Uschi had died tragically two years earlier.

because he spoke English slowly and clearly, making a point of not choosing Anglo-Saxon words when a Romance version existed. This not only communicated what he wanted to say but gave the audience the pleasure of thinking how much their English had improved.

Whilst I went to Montreux, David Duncan arranged to look after Peter during the day as well as the night; I made a timetable for family and friends to come in for company, supper and reading, and flew off in holiday mood. Otto had taken a beautiful room for me in the hotel where the marriage ceremony was to be next day. It overlooked the lake and the mountains and I felt at once refreshed by the surroundings and Otto's kindness.

We had a delicious supper with Alexander and I fell asleep early. Around midnight the telephone rang beside my bed. It was my friend and neighbour Dr. Christine Manning. She told me that Loulie had brought Peter home for lunch and that when he woke, with difficulty, and after a very long sleep, he was very confused and was seeing double. I got up at six next morning and flew home. Peter was very pleased to see me but not surprised, because he wasn't sure that I had gone away.

FOURTEEN

"Not a tragedy, but an epic,"
1985

T HE DOUBLE VISION gradually disappeared, but from that month I began to lose hope that we could get back to the sort of life Peter could enjoy. Three more cerebral attacks shook him, on Christmas Day and in January 1987. He still got pleasure from anything enjoyable and rarely complained, except about my reluctance to give him second helpings.

The last stroke in January took away most of his voice. This was the blow we had always most dreaded. Gradually Peter tried using it again and soon I could understand most of what he wanted to say. We began practising words and sentences with exercises recommended by the speech therapist from the Royal Free Hospital, partly because Peter wanted to talk properly, tired though he was, and partly because he had been invited to perform a ceremony at the University College Zoology Department where he had been professor. The old departments of Zoology and Botany were to become a new Department of Biology, and it had been agreed to give the building Peter's name. I thought Peter should say something flippant, in case there was embarrassment at his performing from a wheelchair. So we practised, "I name this building the Medawar Building," as the plaque was unveiled, and then, "and may God bless all who work in it"—as the Queen used to say when she launched a new ship. We got to the stage of managing the words, but in the end he was too tired, so I stood in for him.

We managed to go to the theatre at New Year with Gayle Hunnicutt and her husband Simon Jenkins. They took a box at the Royalty Theatre where Judy Dench was acting in the play *Mr. and Mrs. Nobody,* based on Grossmith's *Diary of a Nobody.*

Gayle and the manager were waiting outside the theatre. We hauled the wheelchair out of the back of the car, Peter was eased into it and the manager pushed it into the theatre, while I parked the car. Peter couldn't see the finer points of the play, but enough of it to be entertained and to feel part of normal life returning. As we came out of the theatre, it began to snow. Every move we made to get Peter safely into the car and home is fixed in my memory, especially Gayle standing on the pavement with snowflakes catching in her hair, waving and smiling with a mixture of triumph and sadness.

Getting the wheelchair into the house after an evening out was a problem solved by our friend Heinz Wolff, the brilliant bioengineer. He and his team built rails for the wheelchair from the front door down to the street, and fixed a small winch and cable which could be attached to it, both to let it down and to bring it in. I found the procedure rather nerve-racking, especially in the dark, but Peter was trustful and didn't worry.* Sometimes neighbours heard

---

*Even now, he followed his policy of not fretting about a problem unless he himself could do something about it.

the winch turning and came out to help and sometimes passers-by obliged. Peter told me he now had no conception of how our house was arranged, how the rails went or where the street was. After a lot of repetition he got some idea of where he was but it was very hard for him, and heart-breaking to realise what he had lost and what deprivations he was putting up with.

He was very tired. He could not move out of the chair. Before he lost his voice he told a friend that his greatest fear was that he might find himself in front of the television for a "bumper edition of 'The Archers' " and be unable to escape. Actually, in spite of groaning about this series, he did listen and become temporarily entertained. He must have visualised what was going on clearly in his mind or he couldn't have made the joke, because "The Archers" is a radio series.

Although he could barely see, hardly speak or move, he still responded and rarely complained. When the actor Andrew Sachs came to read to him, the right arm was always flung up in greeting and his whole face smiled. When I came in the morning to relieve David Duncan, the arm curved and beckoned me to sit on the side of his chair, where he could put it round me and lift up his face to be kissed. Friends and kisses and wine still gave him pleasure.

Once, he developed a chest infection and had to take a course of antibiotics. Then the invalid's misery of constipation was reversed. One evening when he was already in bed, he signaled to me that he had to go to the bathroom. That night David Duncan was not helping and the substitute nurse and I were not strong enough to get him out of bed and securely into the wheelchair. By the time I had pushed him into the bathroom he had slipped forward and was in danger of slipping right out of the chair. The only possible move was to help him to lie down on the floor. There he lost physical control. Even in this humiliating situation he did not lose his amazing dignity. As we were cleaning everything up, I felt a surge of admiration and compassion. I whispered in his ear,

"I have never loved you more." He smiled again. I half expected to hear him whisper back one of his frequent comments: "R.T.L."— "Rich-tapestry-of-life."

The morning levée took a long time and often Peter fell asleep in the reclining chair as soon as David Duncan had helped him into it. I brought lunch up on a tray; after that he often slept another two hours. Then came what he said was the best time of the day— tea and reading. I re-read *Emma*, George Eliot's *Middlemarch*, and Gordon Haight's biography of George Eliot, and we shared the pleasure. Film on video was another, but smaller pleasure because unless he had seen the film before, his sight could not follow a new scenario. David Attenborough brought us all his *Life on Earth* video tapes and Susan Hampshire sent us *The Forsyte Saga*, in which she had played Fleur Forsyte, and also the TV version of Trollope's Barchester novels.

We had friends to supper six nights out of seven and sometimes seven out of seven. The friends helped to get Peter out of the reclining chair into the wheelchair and down in the lift to the dining room. There the conversation was lively around him and he often made it livelier still. Even when he was tired, and it was so hard for him to eat without spillage, he dominated the party, and on good days his joie de vivre—his familiar "very decided preference for remaining alive"—was infectious and lifted everyone's spirits. Once June Bedford, one of the best of friends, couldn't for a moment remember which President of the United States built Monticello. Peter smiled at her and simply whispered, "Jefferson."

On 27 February we celebrated our fiftieth golden wedding anniversary. We invited fifty friends and relations to a party at home, and Caroline, Charles and his Caroline, and Loulie provided a delicious supper. Alexander and his wife Avis flew in from America with their four-month-old daughter Flora who pleased everybody, including herself, as she was carried from arm to arm.

All over the house there were vases filled with golden flowers—daffodils, freesias, narcissi, azaleas and lilies. The scent reminded me of the Victorian conservatory of my uncle's house where I lived as a child. Caroline had organised a golden wedding cake that was made to look like a book for signatures. It looked so real that two guests got icing on their fingers trying to turn the pages and sign their names.

Peter welcomed friends, two at a time, upstairs, sitting on his bed arranged with cushions like a sofa. Before he got tired we grouped children, grandchildren and cousins round us on the couch for photographs. Some of their eyes glowed like hot coals from the flash, but no child stuck its tongue out and we had a record for the photograph album.

Our last expedition was to the Albert Hall, to listen to a programme that included Brahms's Fourth Symphony. Our friend Richard Frostick had hoped to get us into a box he had been lent, but in spite of every effort by the staff it wasn't possible. Instead, Peter's wheelchair was brought to a narrow platform to one side of and above the orchestra. I sat behind him in a small box from which I could put my hands on his shoulders and tell him what was going on. He conducted the slow movement of the symphony with his left hand and his face showed content.

FIFTEEN

Finale, 1987

D AVID DUNCAN WOKE ME early on the morning of 23
September. "I can't get any response from Sir Peter,"
he said. I ran upstairs and found Peter lying very
quiet in bed. I took his hand and he gave it a slight
squeeze. I knew the only hope was to get him into hospital as fast
as possible.

When John Newsom Davis was appointed Professor of Neurology at Oxford in 1985 he handed Peter's case over to Dr. Peter
Harvey, consultant neurologist at the Royal Free Hospital; it was
so near to us that we could see the top storeys from our house,
behind tall plane trees. I rang the neurology ward at once to ask if
the current shortage of nurses had closed any of their beds. Dr.
Gareth Llewellyn, Dr. Harvey's registrar, answered. He was as

practical and helpful as Peter Harvey himself. Within an hour an ambulance arrived and Peter was in bed in a side room, off the main ward, conscious, but very far away. Peter Harvey came very quickly to see him. We hoped that the effect of whatever damage had occurred in the brainstem might pass, but it didn't. A few days later I noticed that his remaining eye was slewed again to one side, as it had been in New York seven years earlier.

He could still give a wan smile and squeeze my hand, but by 1 October I knew his spirit had gone. All next day his breathing laboured against the rising tide of fluid in his lungs. We stayed with him and I talked to him as if he could hear and be comforted. At nine in the evening of 2 October he died.

We buried Peter in Alfriston Churchyard, on the Sussex Downs. I chose this church because it was near the sea, and a river ran past the wall of the churchyard and down to the sea. Also, this was the one place where I remembered walking with Peter, over the Downs. The vicar, the Reverend John Davey, knew that we were not proper Christians, but having read Peter's books, he and his church wardens welcomed him all the same. We agreed on a simple service. Charles read the lesson for the day. Then Caroline read from Ecclesiastes and I spoke my favourite passage from the last page of Peter's *Hope of Progress*.* As we left the church for the grave, the wind sprang up and a rain cloud burst and soaked us. It made me feel better for a moment because I thought how Peter would have laughed at the dramatic timing.

I had asked that anyone who wanted to give flowers in Peter's memory should instead give a tree through the National Trust. Flowers from his children and me and from the nurses who had looked after him in hospital were waiting by the graveside.

Ten days after Peter's death a hurricane swept over England

---

*This book of essays included the text of Peter's 1969 address to the British Association, entitled "On the Effecting of All Things Possible."

and destroyed 15 million trees. Over £2,500 has so far been sent to the National Trust* in Peter's memory—and even though he hardly knew an oak from an ash, he would be pleased. The damage from fallen trees took months to clear, but by 2 October 1988, the first anniversary of his death, the Medawar Grove was started at Alfriston. A hawthorn and a rowan were planted as the forerunners. Afterwards we held a party for friends, relations, the vicar and representatives of the parish council. I plan to repeat this every year on the first Sunday in October, for everyone who has given a tree.

Ralph Beyer, the sculptor who cut the lettering on the slate tablets round the inner wall of Coventry Cathedral, made the headstone for the grave. Peter's and my names are on it with our birthdays and the date of his death.

The sentence from Thomas Hobbes which he loved is carved at the base of the stone: "There can be no contentment but in proceeding," the last sentence of the lecture he gave at Exeter on the day before his first stroke in 1969.

The words that preceded this sentence are a glorious summary of the beliefs that sustained Peter through his life:

We cannot point to a single definitive solution of any one of the problems that confront us—political, economic, social or moral, that is, having to do with the conduct of life. We are still beginners, and for that reason may hope to improve. To deride the hope of progress is the ultimate fatuity, the last word in poverty of spirit and meanness of mind. There is no need to be dismayed by the fact that we cannot yet envisage a definitive solution of our problems, a resting place beyond which we need not try to go. Because he likened life to a race, and defined felicity as the state of mind of those in the front of it, Thomas Hobbes has always been thought of as the arch materialist, the first man to uphold go-getting as a creed. But this is a travesty of Hobbes' opinion. He was a go-getter in a sense, but it was the going, not the getting he extolled. As Hobbes conceived it, the race had no finishing post. The great thing about the

* National Trust, Queen Annes Gate, London SW1 H9AS

race was to be in it, to be a contestant in the attempt to make the world a better place, and it was a spiritual death he had in mind when he said that to forsake the course is to die. "There is no such thing as perpetual tranquillity of mind while we live here," he told us in *Leviathan*, "because life itself is but motion, and can never be without desire, or without fear no more than without sense. There can be no contentment but in proceeding." I agree.

Postscript

. . . the Grand affair of your life will be to gain and preserve the Friendship and Esteem of your Husband. You are married to a Man of good education and learning, of an excellent understanding, and an exact taste. It is time, and it is happy for you, that these qualities in him are adorned with great Modesty, a most amiable Sweetness of Temper, and an unusual disposition to Sobriety and Virtue: but neither Good Nature nor Virtue will suffer him to esteem you against his Judgement; and although he is not capable of using you ill, yet you will in time grow a thing indifferent and perhaps contemptible; unless you can supply the loss of Youth and Beauty with more durable qualities . . . to become a Reasonable and Agreeable Companion. This must produce in your Husband a true Rational Love and Esteem for you, which old Age will not diminish.

—Jonathan Swift, 1727

PETER WAS STILL ALIVE when I began to write this book, mostly in the afternoons when he was asleep. Of course I told him that I had been invited to write it, and when I read him one of the stories he laughed and approved it—but then forgot. Later, when a friend asked him what he thought of my writing the book, he was astonished, then hesitated, smiled, and said, "The *minx*!"

Peter left hospital and came home in August 1986. Then we still hoped he would improve from the effects of the 1985 stroke—and he did, until June 1987. After that stroke, there could not be much fun for him.

After he died on 2 October 1987, I tried to do what he wanted—and it was what I wanted too. He had said, "If anything should happen to me, you would bash on, wouldn't you?" and I said yes, but without enthusiasm.

In November, my blood pressure rose to 235 over 125; I felt giddy and could hardly walk. Dr. Peter Harvey, who had looked after Peter, told me that I too had had a stroke—fortunately small. I went into the Royal Free Hospital for two weeks' sleep and care and came out almost none the worse.

In December we organised a beautiful memorial service in Westminster Abbey. The Abbey was filled with friends and people who knew Peter—about two thousand in all. Gwyneth Jones sang the "Libera me, Domine" from Verdi's *Requiem*. We had listened to it whenever we could. Peter always claimed that he didn't like what he called "holy music," but this *Requiem* isn't holy in the abnegating mode that displeased him. Loulie organised all the details: the Royal College of Music played, the choir of University College sang, Charles, Caroline and Sir George Porter, the President of the Royal Society, read, and Jim (now Sir James) Gowans spoke about Peter and his life.

At the end, the bells of the Abbey pealed, to lift up our spirits. Somebody said that the service had been very inspiring; somebody else said, "That gave Peter a good send-off."

I was learning that when you lose a loved partner after fifty years, life has to be conducted on the one step after another principle. There are so many things to arrange and to do; you have to get on with them, relying on the friends you knew you had, and on those you didn't know you had. From both sorts, kindness streamed over me. Friends invented reasons to bring me to America, to Germany and to France, sometimes for meetings in Peter's memory and sometimes to travel with the Margaret Pyke Trust Exhibition—"Common Ground International." This linked together the causes of environment, population and relief in ways that encouraged viewers to lend a hand instead of wringing hands in despair.

During the last two years of Peter's life I had found my memory and concentration so unreliable that, like many people well past the halfway mark, I began to wonder if I was starting Alzheimer's disease.

Now, in March 1989, a year and a half after Peter's death, I know that I am not. I am well, busy and sad, but, as Dr. Johnson's old schoolmaster Mr. Edwards said, "Cheerfulness keeps breaking in." When I think of Peter, especially when I look at one of the smiling photographs, a small sudden rush of tears comes into my eyes; but I am gradually forgetting the acid misery of the last hospital days, and remembering all the great things I learnt and gained from Peter. Every time a friend or colleague talks about Peter, they tell me what they "owe" him, how much and how well he influenced them and what fun he gave them. I was lucky to be where I was.

Now that I've finished this book I see how inadequately it paints a picture of Peter, but he was so different from anyone else that he is a very difficult subject to paint, and the times in which we grew up were so astonishingly different from today that our outlook may seem unbelievable to modern couples. Feminists will probably find our attitudes to marriage peculiar. I have described them as they were: they were ours and they worked, even though I often longed for more relaxation en famille, and Peter must often have wished I could play bridge or be more methodical and do less "wondering." I had to stop myself saying, "I wonder what . . ." when he pointed out, early on, that however much I wondered, there wasn't enough material for an answer.

Apart from the consolation of friends, attending to the welfare of the Margaret Pyke Trust, and writing this book, helping David Pyke to select essays for another book by Peter has given me the most backbone and joy.

The book is to be called *The Threat and the Glory* and is to be published by Oxford University Press. It consists of Peter's general essays—mostly written after 1969—chosen out of those printed in various journals but not so far published in book form. They have given us, as they gave him, laughter and delight, and his claim to the best sort of immortality.

Index

Page numbers in *italics* refer to illustrations.